Pocket Guide to
Basic Skills and Procedures

Pocket Guide to
Basic Skills and
Procedures

Anne G. Perry, R.N., M.S.N.

Associate Professor, School of Nursing
St. Louis University
St. Louis, Missouri

Patricia A. Potter, R.N., M.S.N.

Director of Nursing Practice
Barnes Hospital
St. Louis, Missouri

SECOND EDITION

illustrated

The C. V. Mosby Company

St. Louis • Baltimore • Philadelphia • Toronto   1990

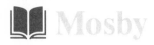

Editor   Nancy L. Coon
Developmental editors   Susan Epstein, Suzanne Seeley
Project manager   Carlotta Seely
Designer   Rey Umali

SECOND EDITION

Copyright © 1990 by The C.V. Mosby Company

Previous edition copyrighted 1986

Printed in the United States of America

The C.V. Mosby Company
11830 Westline Industrial Drive, St. Louis, Missouri 63146

Library of Congress Cataloging in Publication Data

Perry, Anne Griffin.
    Pocket guide to basic skills and procedures / Anne G. Perry,
Patricia A. Potter. — 2nd ed.
        p.   cm.
    Rev. ed. of: Pocket nurse guide to basic skills and procedures.
1986.
    Includes bibliographical references.
    ISBN 0-8016-5527-7
    1. Nursing—Handbooks, manuals, etc.   2. Diagnosis—Handbooks,
manuals, etc.   I. Potter, Patricia Ann.   II. Perry, Anne Griffin.
Pocket nurse guide to basic skills and procedures.   III. Title.
    [DNLM: 1. Nursing—handbooks.   WY 39 P462p]
RT51.P37   1990
610.73—dc20
DNLM/DLC
for Library of Congress   89-13933
                                                              CIP

C/D/D   9   8   7   6   5

Preface

The *Pocket Guide to Basic Skills and Procedures*, second edition, is a quick reference tool for use by both students and practitioners in the clinical setting. It contains 94 skills, many of which nurses will employ on a daily basis in their practice.

Organization

Skills and procedures are grouped according to specialty areas (e.g., medications, fluids, diagnostic procedures). Each skill is presented in an easy-to-read format that includes:

1. The purpose for performing each skill
2. A list of actual or potential nursing diagnoses
3. A list of equipment needed
4. A step-by-step outline of the skill with rationales for every step

The skill concludes with helpful information including nurse alerts, client teaching, and pediatric and geriatric considerations.

Special Features

Because an integral part of any nurse's practice is to formulate nursing diagnoses that will in turn help in planning care for clients, an appendix of approved nursing diagnoses with definitions is provided.

Supplements

Readers are encouraged to refer to Potter-Perry *Fundamentals of Nursing* and Perry-Potter *Clinical Nursing Skills and Techniques* for in-depth discussion of the material presented here.

Anne G. Perry
Patricia A. Potter

Contents

PRELIMINARY SKILLS

Admission into the Health Care System

Whether a client is entering a hospital, a nursing home, or a rehabilitation center, the admission process can be very stressful. It is essential that during the admission process as much information as possible be collected so that the client ultimately receives individualized health care. Inclusion of available friends or family members into the admission process increases their availability to support the client during the experience in the health care setting.

While each institution follows a different set of admission practices, the purposes of admission remain the same. The admission process initiates data collection for nursing care and discharge planning, reduces anxiety and fear, provides an opportunity to teach the client and family, ensures client comfort and safety, and maintains the client's legal rights as a health care recipient.

Potential Nursing Diagnoses

Anxiety related to hospitalization, impending diagnostic and/or treatment procedures, or separation from support persons
Fear related to unknown health status

Equipment

Admission Office

Necessary admitting forms
Identification band
General consent form

Nursing Unit

Personal care items: bed pan and urinal, wash basin, bath towel and washcloth, toiletry items, tissue paper, water pitcher and glass, emesis basin
Assessment forms

Equipment to perform physical assessment: scale, watch with second hand, thermometer, sphygmomanometer, urine collection cup, additional equipment as needed by type of assessment

Steps	Rationale
Admitting Area	
1. Welcome client and escort him and his family to interviewing area.	Reduces anxiety of anticipating first encounter with agency personnel. Interviewing area provides privacy for client.
2. Acquire pertinent identifying information, including client's: Full legal name Age Birthdate Address Next of kin Physician Religion Previous admissions Allergies	Ensures correct legal identification on client's medical records.
3. Apply identification band to client's wrist containing: Client's full legal name Hospital or agency number Physician Birthdate Be sure that band is secure.	Serves as means to officially identify client when therapies or procedures are performed (e.g., medication administration, surgical procedures, x-ray examinations).
4. Instruct client (or legal guardian) to read general consent form for treatment. Assess client's understanding of consent form. ■ Request client (or family member) to sign form if he agrees to be admitted for treatment.	Gives agency right to perform routine procedures and therapies, select room placement, and provide required nursing care.

Steps	Rationale
5. Provide any brochures that describe purpose and organization of agency as well as policies or rules that affect client's conduct.	American Hospital Association's "Patient's Bill of Rights" states that client must have access to this information.
6. Assign a room on basis of client's condition, health care needs, and personal preferences.	Clients requiring frequent observation and therapy should be close to central nursing station. Consideration of client's personal preferences during room selection minimizes anxiety and prevents conflict with other clients. Room environment can provide sensory stimulation for sensorially deprived clients.
7. Direct client to area where technicians in admitting office will collect routine blood specimens and perform chest x-ray and electrocardiographic examinations.	Routine diagnostic testing serves to screen clients for presence of common physical alterations.
instruct client on method for collecting urine specimen.	Specimen may be collected in admitting area or on nursing division.
8. Notify nursing division of client's admission. ■ Report client's name, assigned room and bed, admitting physician, diagnosis, and pertinent information relating to client's condition (e.g., IV line infusing, need for oxygen).	Allows nursing personnel to prepare room and obtain necessary equipment for client's arrival. Client may be admitted directly from emergency room.
9. Transport client and family members to nursing division, using an escort.	Promotes timely and safe arrival to nursing division.

Steps	Rationale
10. On nursing division, introduce client and his family to nurse who is assuming client's care.	Provides client a sense of personalization during admission process.
11. Share with nursing staff pertinent observations about client's behaviors or level of knowledge regarding need for health care.	Promotes continuity of care so nursing staff can assist client in coping with new environment and procedures of care.

Nursing Division

Steps	Rationale
1. Wash hands.	Prevents spread of microorganisms.
2. Prepare assigned room with necessary equipment and personal care items.	Availability of equipment for personal care promotes client comfort by preventing unnecessary delays during care delivery.
3. Prepare client's bed by adjusting it to lowest horizontal position. Turn down top sheet and spread.	Makes it easier and safer for client to get into bed.
4. Greet client and his family cordially. Introduce yourself by name and job title, telling client you are responsible for his care.	Reduces anxiety client may feel regarding admission. Awareness of which nurse is responsible for his care expedites requests client may have.
5. Escort client and family members to assigned room. Introduce them to roommate if semiprivate room is assigned.	Orientation begins with introduction to roommate.
6. Assess client's general appearance, noting signs or symptoms of physical distress.	If client is experiencing any acute physical problems, routine admission procedures should be postponed until these are cared for.

Steps	Rationale
7. Check physician's orders for any treatment measures that should be initiated immediately.	Delay in initiation of therapies can cause worsening of client's condition.
8. Assess client's and family member's psychological status by noting nonverbal behaviors and verbal responses to greetings and explanations.	Client's level of anxiety influences his ability to adapt to health care environment.
9. Orient client to nursing division:	Promotes understanding of agency policies and procedures.
■ Introduce staff members who enter room.	
■ Explain who head nurse or clinical nurse of division is and that person's role in solving problems.	
■ Explain visiting hours and their purpose.	Family members' willingness to follow visiting hour policy ensures that client will receive adequate rest.
■ Discuss smoking policy.	
■ Demonstrate how to use equipment in room (e.g., bed, over-bed table, lighting).	Client safety depends on understanding of policies and how to use equipment correctly.
■ Show client how to use nurse call light.	
■ Escort client to bathroom (if able to ambulate).	
■ Explain hours for meal time and nourishments.	
■ Describe services available (e.g., chaplain visitation, gift shop, activity therapy).	
■ Explain areas where client and family might visit (e.g., cafeteria, lounge, recreation room).	

Steps	Rationale
■ Warn client against keeping large sums of money or valuables in own room in agency ■ Inform client about procedure for acquiring television or radio.	Because clients are often required to leave their rooms during day, there is risk of money or valuables being stolen.
10. Collect any valuables client wishes to have placed in agency safe. Place articles in specially labeled and sealed envelope. Instruct client to sign statement releasing agency of responsibility for valuables.	Protects client from theft.
11. Explain to client that admitting process will include a nursing history and physical examination. Request client to change into appropriate gown. Provide privacy.	Keeping client informed of procedures and their purpose minimizes anxiety. Hospital gown or pajamas makes it easier to expose body parts during examination.
12. Assist client with hanging or storing clothing in closet or locker.	Basic to most person's self-image is keeping personal items neat and properly stored.
13. If client prefers, family members may stay in room during history taking; otherwise, escort family to waiting area.	Client may be embarrassed by sharing personal information about his health with family members.
14. Wash hands.	Reduces transmission of microorganisms.
15. Prepare equipment for nursing history and assessment.	Prevents delays that might increase client's anxiety or fatigue.
16. Weigh client and record his height.	Determines baseline values and any recent change in weight.
17. Assist client to assume comfortable position in bed or in bedside chair.	Relieves anxiety and thereby increases accuracy of findings.

Steps	Rationale
18. Assess client's vital signs.	Provides baseline measurement to compare with future findings and discloses any alterations from normal expected range.
19. Obtain nursing history:	Provides data necessary to develop individualized plan of care based on client's identified health problems.
Client's perceptions of illness	
Past medical history	
Presenting signs and symptoms	
Risk factors for illness	
History of allergies (Nurse provides client an allergy band, similar in size to an identification band, that lists all foods, drugs, or substances to which client is allergic.)	Alerts nurses to substances to which client is allergic. Prevents accidental administration of substances when client is confused or nonresponsive.
Medication history (If client brings medications to agency, nurse instructs him to take them home; otherwise, medications are stored on division for safekeeping.)	Therapeutic drug administration depends on correct dosages and proper timing as well as avoidance of drug incompatibilities.
Alterations in activities of daily living	Identifying client and family needs early helps in planning for eventual discharge from agency.
Family resources and support	
Potential risk factors affecting discharge planning	
Client's knowledge of health problems and implications for long-term care.	Allows nurse to plan for necessary instruction to prepare client for eventual discharge.
20. Conduct physical assessment of appropriate body systems.	Provides objective data for identifying client's health problems.

Steps	Rationale
21. Instruct client on proper technique to provide urine specimen. (If not obtained in admitting.) ■ Label specimen and attach requisition form.	Urinalysis is a basic test to screen for renal and metabolic problems, fluid and electrolyte alterations, and lower urinary tract alterations.
22. Explain to client that technicians will be obtaining blood specimens and performing chest x-ray and electrocardiographic examinations (if not performed in admitting office).	CBC is routine test used to screen for anemias. Blood typing and cross-match are necessary for clients undergoing surgery or who are expected to receive blood transfusions. Chest x-ray screens for preexisting lung disease. Electrocardiogram screens for conduction defects of heart.
23. Inform client about any planned procedures or treatments scheduled for next shift or day (e.g., visit by physician, additional x-rays, dietary restrictions).	Client has right to be informed of any procedures or treatments that he will undergo. Being able to anticipate planned therapies minimizes anxiety.
24. Provide client opportunity to ask questions about any procedure or therapies.	Helps clarify any misconceptions.
25. Allow client and family time together alone.	Admission procedure can be stressful and fatiguing. Client and family often have decisions to make or concerns to share before visitation ends.
26. Be sure call light is within reach, bed is in low position, and side rails are raised.	Provides for client safety.
27. Wash hands.	Reduces transmission of microorganisms.
28. Record history and assessment findings on appropriate forms.	Prompt and thorough documentation prevents deletion of data.

Steps	Rationale
29. Notify physician of client's admission and report any unusual findings.	Client's condition may require immediate medical intervention.
30. Begin to develop nursing care plan.	Provides for continuity of individualized care.

Nurse Alert

When a critically ill client reaches a hospital's nursing division, extensive examination, diagnostic procedures, and treatment procedures become necessary almost immediately. Time constraints may force the nurse to delay certain steps in the admission process.

Client Teaching

Teaching can occur during the admission process. A nurse can provide information regarding physical assessment findings, planned diagnostic procedures, or hospital routines. A formal teaching plan is designed and implemented after a nursing assessment and care plan are completed.

Pediatric Considerations

Thorough explanation of the hospital experience and related procedures will reduce a child's fear of the unknown. Ideally children should be prepared for hospitalization before admission, either by parents or by the nursing staff. A tour of hospital facilities and the use of dolls, puppet shows, or specially produced children's films to demonstrate procedures are techniques that will help the child understand hospitalization.

Geriatric Considerations

An elderly person who is to be admitted into a long-term care facility or nursing home often undergoes extensive screening. When such a person enters the hospital, it is very important to orient him to his new surroundings. Gradual loss of sensory perception places the elderly client at risk of sensory overload, resulting in confusion or feelings of isolation.

Making a Referral
for Health Care
Services

Often clients require services of various departments within an agency or services from a different facility altogether. The nurse frequently recognizes the need for additional resources and initiates the referral process. Whatever type of referral is needed, it is important that the nurse collaborate with members of other disciplines so that the clients' individual needs are met.

The purposes of the referral process are to provide the clients with expert services the nurse or the physician cannot provide, to improve the continuity of care throughout the client discharge and return to the home, and, last, to adequately prepare the client for discharge.

Potential Nursing Diagnoses

Knowledge deficit regarding therapy related to inexperience
Anxiety related to new personnel/agency
Self-care deficit related to physical restriction
Impaired verbal communication related to hearing loss

Steps	Rationale
1. Assess client's need for services from other hospital departments. Consider clients' current and posthospital needs.	Other health professionals specialize in skills and knowledge that afford clients services the nurse often cannot offer.

:

11

Steps	Rationale
a. Dietary—recognize factors such as client's repeated intolerance to diet, weight loss, or verbalized discontent with food choices. Client may express poor understanding of newly prescribed diet or diet restrictions.	Registered dietitian can determine nutrients and food sources clients require, based on clients' physical condition. Dietitian has educational aides available to teach about diets.
b. Social work—assess client's need for counseling for major crises, e.g., terminal illness, loss of body part, family problems, need for relocation after discharge to nursing home or extended care facilities; financial resources to cover medical costs; equipment for home health care; transport home following discharge.	Social worker is qualified to conduct regular counseling sessions with clients needing some assistance to cope with life crises. Social workers are also knowledgeable of many resources in community to help client with health care problems.
c. Physical therapy—assess client's need for regular exercise and mobility training following injury, surgery, or as result of chronic illness. Consider length of client's potential rehabilitation period.	Physical therapist is licensed to assist in examination and treatment of physically disabled or handicapped persons. Therapist assists in rehabilitating clients and restoring normal function.
d. Occupational therapy—assess client's need to learn new vocational skills or techniques to perform activities of daily living, following a disability resulting from injury or illness.	Occupational therapists train clients to adapt to physical handicaps by learning new vocational skills or activities of daily living.

Steps	Rationale
e. Speech therapy—assess client's ability to communicate, which has been altered as result of surgery, injury, or illness.	Speech therapist is trained to assist client with disorders affecting normal oral communication.
f. Home health services—assess client's need for intermittent skilled nursing care or physical/speech therapy following discharge.	Home health nurses can provide a follow-up visit as well as regular and frequent nursing services (e.g., administration of injections, wound care, ostomy care). This can help to shorten a client's length of stay in a hospital.
2. Obtain necessary order for referral and communicate with appropriate department client's specific health care needs that will influence therapies. (When order is not needed, nurse may confer directly with health care provider.)	Department accepting referral will require basic information about client before visits begin. Information related to nursing care needs may influence type of therapy referral service provides.
3. Explain to client that therapist from another department will be visiting.	Client has right to know of proposed treatment measures.
4. Consult with referral service about nursing implications related to prescribed treatments (e.g., exercises, diet restrictions, communication techniques).	Therapies initiated by referral service may pose implications for type and extent of care nurse delivers.
5. Determine extent to which client's needs are met by referral service, e.g., has client's dietary intake improved or has weight gain occurred? Is client's range of motion or motor strength improving? Is client learning alternative communication techniques?	Nurse is in best position to judge efficacy of care and coordinate all available resources. Continuing problems may indicate need for different referral or adjustment in nursing care plan.

Steps	Rationale
6. Record information regarding type of referral and frequency of visits in Kardex and care plan.	Provides continuity of care.

Nurse Alert

Availability of services varies according to size and type of health care agency. In many agencies multidisciplinary team conferences provide excellent opportunity for discussing client's needs and making referrals.

Client Teaching

The client needs to be taught the specifics about the role of each new therapist who is introduced into the care activities. Likewise if the client is going to be receiving these services in the home environment, the nurse needs to educate the client about the anticipated services and how the client may contact the service provider directly.

Pediatric Considerations

Referrals for pediatric clients may include the siblings as well as the child's parents. In addition, the child's developmental needs and physiological and psychosocial needs are considered when initiating referrals.

Geriatric Considerations

The needs of the older adult vary with any cognitive and physical impairments present. Some services for the older adult can include day care activities and other social services in the areas of nutritional support, transportation, and safety.

Discharge from a Health Care Agency

Successful discharge planning is a coordinated interdisciplinary process that ensures that all clients have a plan for continuing care after they leave the hospital (AHA, 1983). The client's discharge should come as a surprise to no one.

In 1985, the Society for Hospital Social Work Directors of the American Hospital Association described four levels of outcomes for clients at discharge: (1) client and family understanding of the diagnosis, anticipated level of function, discharge medications, and anticipated medical follow-up; (2) specialized instruction or training so that the client or family can provide posthospital care; (3) coordination of community support systems that enable the client to return home; and (4) relocation of the client and coordination of support systems or transfer to another health care facility. Typically nurses are actively involved in assisting clients with the first and second outcomes while social workers manage the third and fourth. However, in many institutions a nurse may be the one individual to coordinate the efforts of all health team members in meeting each of the outcomes. If the client's need for discharge planning is identified early during a hospital stay, there is a greater likelihood for mutual goal setting with the client and family and a realistic discharge plan.

Potential Nursing Diagnoses

Bathing/hygiene self-care deficit related to physical restrictions
Knowledge deficit regarding health care practices related to lack of experience
Potential for injury related to environmental barriers in the home
Anxiety related to impending discharge

Equipment

Necessary instructional materials
Any ordered prescriptions
Discharge summary form
Utility cart
Wheelchair

Steps	Rationale
Day of Admission	
1. Assess client's health care needs for discharge. Use nursing history, care plan, and ongoing assessments.	The plan for discharge begins at admission and continues throughout course of a client's stay in the agency. It facilitates eventual adjustment to home setting.
2. Assess client's and family members' needs for health teaching related to therapies to be administered at home, restrictions resulting from health alterations, and complications.	Client's and family's understanding of health care needs will improve likelihood of successfully achieving self-care at home. Inclusion of family members in teaching sessions provides client with an available resource when at home.
3. Evaluate with client and family any environmental factors in home setting that might interfere with self-care activities.	Environmental barriers may pose risks to client's safety as result of limitation created by client's illness or need for certain therapies.
4. Assess client's acceptance of health problems and related restrictions.	Client's acceptance of health status can affect his willingness to adhere to therapies and/or restrictions after discharge.
5. Consult with other health team members (e.g., dietitian, social worker) regarding client's needs on discharge.	Members of all health care disciplines should collaborate to determine client's needs and functional abilities.

Steps	Rationale
6. Collaborate with physician in assessing need for referral to skilled home health agencies.	Clients eligible for home health care are confined to home as a result of illness, are under a physician's supervision, or require skilled nursing care on an intermittent basis.
7. Ask client or family members for suggestions on ways to prepare for discharge.	Client should become part of discharge planning team. He may be able to identify additional needs for support or resources that your assessment did not reveal.
8. Suggest methods for altering physical arrangement of home environment to meet client's needs.	Client's level of independence can be maintained within an environment conducive to his safety and ability to retain function. Advanced preparation may be needed before client actually returns home.
9. Offer client and family information about community health care resources.	Community resources often include services that client or family cannot provide.
10. Conduct teaching sessions with client and family as soon as possible during hospitalization on such topics as: Signs and symptoms of complications Injections, wound care, transfer techniques, colostomy care Medications, diet, exercise Restrictions imposed by illness or surgery	Gives client and family opportunities to practice new skills, ask questions about therapies, and obtain necessary feedback from you to ensure that learning has occurred.

Steps	Rationale
11. Complete any referral forms indicating client's health care needs as well as existing functional abilities.	Continuity of health care is ensured through communication of individualized plan to all health team members.

Day of Discharge

Steps	Rationale
1. Provide client and family an opportunity to ask questions or discuss issues related to health care needs at home.	Allows for final clarification of information previously discussed. Helps relieve client's anxiety.
2. Check physician's discharge orders for prescriptions, change in treatments, or need for special appliances.	Discharge is authorized only by physician. Early check of orders permits attention to any last-minute treatments or procedures in advance of actual discharge.
3. Determine if client or family member has arranged for transport home.	Client's condition at discharge will determine method for transport home.
4. Offer assistance as client dresses into own clothes and packs all personal belongings. Provide privacy as needed.	Promotes client comfort.
5. Make a final check of closets and drawers to be sure that all of client's belongings have been removed.	Prevents loss of client's personal items.
6. Obtain copy of valuables list signed by client at admission and have security personnel or appropriate administrator deliver valuables to client. Have client put initials on receipt.	Client's signature on list will verify receipt of items.
7. Be sure that all valuables are accounted for.	Relieves agency of liability for any losses.

Steps	Rationale
8. Check that client has any prescriptions or medications ordered by physician. Review with him and a family member drug dosage and precautions as well as other pertinent information.	Review of drug information provides feedback to determine client's success in learning about medications.
9. Contact agency's business office to determine if client needs to finalize arrangements for payment of bill. Arrange for client or family member to visit office.	A source of concern for many clients is whether agency has accepted insurance or other payment forms.
10. Acquire utility cart to move client's belongings. Obtain wheelchair for clients unable to ambulate. Clients leaving by ambulance will be transported on ambulance stretchers.	Provides for safe transport.
11. Use proper body mechanics and transfer techniques in assisting client to wheelchair or stretcher.	Prevents injury to you and to client.
12. Escort client to entrance of agency where source of transportation is waiting.	Agency policy requires escort to ensure client's safe exit.
13. Lock wheelchair wheels. Assist client in transferring to automobile or transport vehicle. Help family member place personal belongings inside vehicle.	Agency's liability ends once client is safely in vehicle.
14. Return to division and notify admitting or appropriate department of time client was discharged.	Allows agency to prepare for admission of next client.
15. Complete discharge summary in clients' medical record.	Essential for documenting client's status at time of departure from agency.

Nurse Alert

Do not ignore clients who fail to pose an obvious need for discharge planning. Too often clients with short stays in a health care agency may not receive teaching or necessary referrals until the day of discharge.

Client Teaching

Individualize any discussions or demonstrations so the client can easily apply what he learns to the home setting.

Pediatric Considerations

A child's developmental age must be considered before attempting to prepare him for any home-care skills. Parents are most commonly involved in any preparation for the child's discharge.

Geriatric Considerations

Elderly clients with mobility restrictions or sensory limitations will benefit from the installation of safety and/or assistive devices (such as grab bars around toilets, new lighting in bathrooms, or chair height adjustments to make bending easier).

Writing a Nursing
Diagnosis

A nursing diagnosis is a statement of the client's potential or actual health problem that the nurse is licensed and competent to treat. The overall purpose of the nursing diagnosis is to interpret assessment data and thus identify health problems involving the client, the family, and significant others.

The diagnostic process includes three major elements: analysis and interpretation of data, identification of client problems, and formulation of nursing diagnoses.

1. Analysis and interpretation of data require data validation and data clustering. Validation involves determining the relationship between assessment data and health needs and determining their accuracy. Data clustering is the process that the nurse uses to group related data.

2. Identification of client problems involves determining what the general health problems are and whether they are actual or potential problems. When identifying client needs the nurse must consider all aspects of the nursing assessment.

3. Formulation of actual nursing diagnoses identifies the specific nursing care need of each client. Individualization of such needs allows the nurse to develop a specific nursing care plan for each of her clients.

Clients entering a health care agency may have more than one nursing diagnosis based on their individual health care problem. The Appendix, at the end of this text, includes the nursing diagnoses currently accepted by the North American Nursing Diagnosis Association (NANDA).

Steps	Rationale
1. Validate pertinent data identified during history taking and physical assessment. Validation can be achieved from secondary source of information such as client, reexamination, or results of laboratory tests.	Determines whether data gathered during assessment are complete and accurate.

EXAMPLE
Client states he gets short of breath climbing stairs. *Data validation:* Client is requested to climb stairs in his home. After climbing six stairs, he shows respiratory rate increase from 18 to 32 breaths/min. Nasal flaring and diaphoresis are present, pulse rate is increased from 82 to 126. BP is stable at 130/82.

Steps	Rationale
2. Group related data, which are generally signs and symptoms indicating general health problem. Related data are clustered as regards client's mental or emotional status, individual body systems, risk factors, family data, and community factors.	Clustering of data encourages you to identify patterns for health care. Data clustering groups defining characteristics from the nursing health history and ultimately leads to formation of nursing diagnoses.

EXAMPLE
Client states that he has shortness of breath with exertion. *Data clustering:* Respiratory rate is increased from 18 to 32 breaths/min. Pulse rate is increased from 82 to 126 with exertion. Nasal flaring and diaphoresis are present with exertion.

Steps	Rationale
3. List general health care problems of client. a. Actual health care problem: one that is currently perceived by client b. Potential health care problem: one that client is at risk of developing	Allows beginning nurse to identify broad general nursing problems.

EXAMPLE
- *Actual* health care problem—shortness of breath with exertion
- *Potential* health care problem—reduced activity level

4. Write nursing diagnosis in two parts. a. Problem: actual or potential client need that can be resolved by nursing interventions	Nursing diagnostic label (NANDA).
b. Cause: direct or contributing factor in development of client need	Helps to individualize nursing diagnosis and subsequent plan of care.

EXAMPLE
- *Problem*—ineffective breathing pattern related to *cause* (exertion)
- *Problem*—potential activity intolerance related to *cause* (shortness of breath)

5. Reevaluate list of individualized nursing diagnoses developed for each client contact.	As client's needs change, nursing diagnoses are modified. Some may no longer be relevant, while new ones may need to be developed.

Writing a Nursing Care Plan

The nursing care plan is a written guideline for client care so the specifics of nursing care can be quickly communicated to all nursing personnel. Written nursing care plans document the individual health care needs of the client as determined by assessment and the nursing diagnoses. During planning, priorities, goals, and expected outcomes are formulated to coordinate nursing care, promote continuity of care, and list criteria that will be used in the evaluation of nursing care. In addition, the written care plan communicates to other nurses and health professionals specific individualized nursing therapies.

Steps	Rationale
1. Determine client centered goals of nursing care for each nursing diagnosis.	Goal is specific aim planned to assist client in achieving maximum level of wellness. Setting goals is an activity that includes family and significant others, as well as the client. Ultimately it determines the expected outcome of the nursing intervention.

EXAMPLE

Nursing diagnoses	Goals
Ineffective coping related to fear of medical diagnosis	Mr. Brown assumes responsibility for seeking support resources
Ineffective airway clearance postoperatively related to abdominal incision	Mr. Brown's lungs to remain clear postoperatively

Steps	Rationale
2. Establish priorities of care. Rank nursing diagnoses and goals in order of importance. Priorities are classified as high, intermediate, or low.	High-priority nursing diagnoses reflect emergency or immediate needs of client. High priorities occur in psychological as well as psychological dimensions. Intermediate-priority nursing diagnoses reflect nonemergency non-life-threatening needs of client. Low-priority nursing diagnoses reflect client goals not directly related to his specific illness or prognosis.

EXAMPLE

Nursing diagnoses	*Rationale for priority setting*
High Priority	
Ineffective coping related to fear of medical diagnosis of cancer	Dealing with this early will help Mr. Brown prepare for surgery and his postoperative restorative care.
Ineffective airway clearance postoperatively related to abdominal incision	Because of this, you will institute preventive client education preoperatively.
Intermediate Priority	
Diarrhea related to unknown cause	Does not affect client's immediate physiological or emotional status. Also, future surgery will assist you in resolving diagnosis.
Low Priority	
Potential infection related to airway secretions	Reflects long-term needs of client.
3. For each nursing diagnosis, write expected outcomes anticipated from nursing action. Outcomes should reflect goals established in Step 1.	Change in client's condition that care plan is designed to bring about. Includes degree of wellness and need for continuing care, medications, support, counseling, and education.

Steps	Rationale

EXAMPLE

Nursing diagnosis
   Ineffective airway clearance
   postoperatively related to
   abdominal incision

Goal	*Expected outcome*
Mr. Brown's lungs to remain clear postoperatively	Lungs clear to auscultation
4. Write specific implementation measures. Should include when, how much, where, etc.	Must be specific so there is continuity of care from one nurse to another.
5. Modify nursing care plan based on nursing evaluation of client's status or needs change.	Continually individualizes nursing care for client based on his changing needs.

Communicating during the Orientation Phase

Communication is the means to understanding and caring for the client. Without effective communication skills the nurse is often ineffective with the care she provides. Communication skills are a vital part of every interaction that goes on between nurse and client. When effective communication is practiced and integrated into the nurse's care, it becomes a powerful tool in all aspects of nursing.

This skill can be useful to the nurse in the process of planned purposeful communication with a client. It reviews the basic steps used during the orientation phase of the nurse-client relationship. It is important to remember that a nurse's interaction may be brief or long and may require different techniques depending on the purpose or situations involved in the interaction. Any communication with a client must be through a relationship based on mutual trust so a meaningful interaction occurs.

Potential Nursing Diagnoses

Anxiety related to hospitalization, impending surgery, separation from family

Fear related to impending surgery or therapy

Knowledge deficit regarding hospitalization related to limited experience with illness

Impaired verbal communication related to:
  Sensory deficit
  Different culture/language
  Surgical procedures, e.g., tracheostomy

Steps	Rationale
1. Determine type and availability of environment most conducive to interaction:	Certain environments are more conducive to therapeutic interactions than others.

Steps	Rationale
■ Choose private environment for certain tasks and interactions (e.g., discussion of planned therapy, fear of death, concerns over family members).	Privacy is less threatening to client. Promotes freer expression of feelings.
2. Reduce or eliminate sources of distraction or interruptions in environment.	Ongoing activity, loud noises, and interruptions may hinder message that was intended.
3. Take care of client's physical discomfort or needs before beginning discussion (e.g., positioning, liquids or food, pain relief, assistance to bathroom).	Decreases client's distraction.
4. Create initial climate of warmth and acceptance:	Facilitates more open exchange.
■ Decrease your own anxiety by preparing for interaction, pausing and collecting thoughts before entering room, relaxing by taking several deep breaths.	Helps decrease client's anxiety by seeing you in calm relaxed state.
5. Sit in comfortable chair near client. Make sure that you are at same eye level, facing each other and maintaining good eye contact.	Physical attending provides nonverbal message to client that you are interested in him.
■ Maintain "open" position (avoid crossing your legs and arms), leaning toward client and remaining relatively relaxed.	Demonstrates willingness to communicate.

Steps	Rationale
6. Listen to or observe client's nonverbal behavior. (This often carries emotional dimension of messages.) Listen to client's verbal behavior. Take time to listen. Teach yourself to concentrate. Don't interrupt. Listen "between the lines."	Psychological attending makes you more alert to client's true message. It is also congruent with your nonverbal message conveyed in physical attending.
7. Introduce yourself and provide information:	Assists in orientation.
■ About hospital or agency facilities and environment (e.g., call light, bed adjustments, cabinet space, special equipment).	Increases client's capability of managing environment.
■ Give any informational pamphlets (e.g., orientation to area of care, services available, treatment and/or testing procedures).	Reinforces teaching and allows client to review material.
■ About plan of care (e.g., procedures that need to be completed, activities, gathering specimens).	Increases client's participation in care because of better understanding.
■ Provide general schedule for day.	Helps both you and client plan day or alter schedule.
8. Help client manage anxiety by providing information regarding what he can expect, checking on and acknowledging him frequently, encouraging him to participate in usual activities as much as possible, assisting him in expressing concerns and fears.	In orientation phase anxiety may be related to fear of unknown or changes and interruptions in usual activities or lifestyle.

Steps	Rationale
9. Use communication techniques and tools that facilitate orientation phase:	Assists in establishing rapport with client that promotes free exchange of information.
■ *Accurate empathy*. Listen to message. Respond frequently but briefly to message; respond to both feelings and content. Attend carefully to signs that either confirm or deny accuracy of your response.	Communicates understanding of client's feelings and experiences. Client senses your interest in what he has to say.
■ *Respect*. Be "for" the client. Be willing and available to work with him. Recognize his uniqueness. Practice psychological and physical attending. Suspend critical judgments. Express warmth. Give recognition by greeting client or indicate awareness of change or efforts being made by client.	Communicates positive regard for client.
■ *Genuineness*. Be nondefensive. Be consistent in what you think, feel, and say. Be spontaneous but not impulsive. Avoid facade.	You must be basically yourself and allow client to be himself.
■ *Concreteness*. Do not let client ramble. Ask for more specific information. Avoid vagueness ("I noticed that you have been staying in your bed today"). Begin to explore ("Tell me more about . . ."). Clarification ("I'm not sure I follow."). Paraphrase or restate client's message.	By speaking about specific experiences, specific behaviors, and/or specific feelings, client is likely to speak of specific problems with specific solutions.

Steps	Rationale
10. Use questions carefully:	
■ Use open-ended and nonthreatening questions as much as possible.	Client is usually more willing to express himself.
■ Avoid numerous direct questions; avoid using why and how as much as possible.	Numerous direct questions and why and how questions can be intimidating and annoying to client.
11. Avoid communication breakdown in orientation phase, caused by:	This occurs when message is not received, or is distorted, or is not understood.
Rushing into working phase before establishment of initial trust and rapport.	Client may not be ready and may resist working with you.
Uncomfortable silence.	Increases client's anxiety.
Your anxiety increasing with client's anxiety.	May hinder development of trust and confidence.
Vagueness in answering client's questions.	Client may begin to lack confidence in your ability.
12. Summarize with client what has been discussed during interaction:	Signals close of interaction, allows you and client to depart with same idea, and provides sense of closure at completion of discussion.
"Let me see if I have everything we talked about. We reviewed your treatment plan and what you will need to do. You expressed concern about your length of stay at the hospital and not being able to return to work immediately. Is there anything else?"	
13. Record in nurse's notes communication pertinent to client's health, responses to illness or therapies, and acceptance of health care measures.	Provides data for assessment of client's needs and problems.

Steps	Rationale
■ Include behaviors or non-verbal cues that reflect client's refusal or acceptance of health care measures and response toward therapies.	Documents client's response to nursing care.

Nurse Alert

Throughout any discussion with a client it is important for the nurse to observe his nonverbal behavioral responses. Nonverbal feedback reveals the client's willingness to communicate and can help the nurse redirect communication when the interaction is faltering.

Client Teaching

Effective communication is essential for any form of client education. While the nurse attempts to establish a relationship with a client, she can also determine his readiness and ability to learn.

Pediatric Considerations

A nurse must be able to communicate effectively not only with a child but with the child's parents as well. Nonverbal communication tends to convey the most significant messages to children. Children are very alert to a nurse's feelings, attitudes, and anxiety. The nurse must establish a sense of trust with the child. A quiet, unhurried, and confident voice works best with children of any age.

Geriatric Considerations

When communicating with elderly clients, remember that they bring a world of experiences with them. Aging does not automatically impair intelligence or insight. The nurse will have to adjust communication techniques for those clients with sensory or perceptual alterations (for example, reduced hearing or vision, poor attention span, impaired memory).

Communicating with the Anxious Client

It is quite common for a nurse to encounter a client who is experiencing anxiety. A newly diagnosed illness, separation from family, the discomfort of diagnostic and/or treatment procedures, the threat of surgery, and the expectations of life changes are examples of factors that can cause a client to become anxious. How effectively the nurse can communicate with a client will affect the extent to which his anxiety can be relieved. The purpose of the communication methods in this skill can assist the nurse in helping an anxious client clarify the factors causing anxiety and cope with anxiety-producing situations more effectively.

Potential Nursing Diagnoses

Anxiety related to alterations in life-style
Impaired verbal communication related to anxiety
Ineffective individual coping related to impending surgery or diagnostic findings

Steps	Rationale
1. Provide quiet calm environment, away from groups of people and activity.	Decreasing stimuli can have a calming result.
2. Allow ample personal space.	There is direct correlation between amount of personal space needed and level of anxiety. Nature of nurse-client relationship may determine personal space needed.
3. Acknowledge and take care of anxious client's physical and emotional discomfort but avoid dwelling on physical complaints.	Anxiety can be very unpleasant emotional experience and sometimes is expressed in physical discomfort or complaints.

Steps	Rationale
4. Create climate of warmth and acceptance:	Can have calming effect on client.
■ Maintain composure during interaction.	
■ Stay with client or check frequently if he is experiencing extreme anxiety.	Provides reassurance to anxious client.
■ Demonstrate genuineness and respect.	Allows client to be himself and creates attitude that communicates positive regard between you and client.
5. Use physical attending:	Nonverbal message to client conveys your interest.
■ Sit in comfortable chair near client.	
■ Maintain same eye level with client, facing him. Maintain "open" position (avoid crossing your legs and arms), leaning toward client and remaining relaxed.	
6. Use psychological attending:	Enables you to be more alert to client's message.
■ Listen to client's verbal behavior. Take time to listen; concentrate. Don't interrupt; listen "between the lines"	
7. Provide brief simple introduction: introduce yourself and state who you are. Explain purpose of interaction.	Anxiety may limit amount of information client can understand.
8. Use communication techniques and tools to respond to an anxious client:	
■ Anticipate needs.	Client may ignore his needs. Meeting needs makes him more comfortable.

Steps	Rationale
■ Make replies simple, clear, and related to situation.	Client's perception and attention may be limited.
■ Avoid introducing anything new.	Client may become overwhelmed by new situation or experience.
■ Limit amount of decision making.	Prevents further escalation of anxiety.
■ Provide for physical activity, such as walking.	Requires little concentration and can help decrease anxiety.
■ Use accurate empathy. State what you understand message to be (e.g., "I understand you to say . . ."; "I hear you saying . . ."; "I sense that . . .").	Communicating understanding often has a de-escalating effect on anxiety.
■ Use concreteness.	Can often eliminate vagueness associated with anxiety.
9. Use questions and responses based on hierarchy: description of experience, thoughts about experience, feelings that experience generates:	Aids client in describing event and clarifying his thoughts and feelings.

Nurse: What happened? I sense that you are upset about something.

Client: The doctor was just here. (Describes experience)

Nurse: Tell me more about what happened. (Offers to explore experience further)

Client: He said I won't be getting to go home tomorrow and that I will have to stay until I am able to eat more.

Steps	Rationale
Nurse: What do you think about that? (Requests thoughts about experience)	
Client: Well, I know he is right. I haven't been eating, but I was counting on going home.	
Nurse: What are your feelings? (Offers to explore the experience further)	
Client: I'm disappointed and angry, but I need to stay here for now.	
10. Don't let communication breakdown occur with anxious client: belittling thoughts and feelings associated with anxiety (e.g., "There is no reason why you should feel this way"); ignoring his discomfort connected with anxiety; ignoring him; getting angry with him (e.g., "You have to stop this right now!"); being unable to acknowledge and control your own anxiety.	Communication breakdown can increase anxiety and feelings of isolation.
11. Record in nurse's notes cause of client's anxiety and any exhibited signs and symptoms or behaviors:	Documents nature of client's problem and his response.
■ Include methods used to relieve anxiety and client's response.	Provides guidelines for other nurses to continue interaction.

Nurse Alert

The nurse's interaction can increase a client's anxiety if techniques are not used appropriately. Be alert for signs of anxiety. Physical signs can include dry mouth, sweaty palms, diarrhea, urinary frequency, increases in the respiratory and heart rate and in blood pressure, headache, nausea, and upset stomach. Behavioral signs of anxiety can include tense voice, difficulty in concentrating, insomnia, loss of appetite, pacing, inability to sit still, wringing of hands, expanding one aspect of the total situation out of proportion, and irritability.

Client Teaching

Teaching should not be conducted when a client is anxious. He will then likely be unable to attend to your instructions.

Pediatric Considerations

Communicate at the child's level by sitting on a low chair, kneeling, squatting, or even sitting on the floor. Preserve physical closeness with the parent if possible by allowing the child to sit on the parent's lap. Use of dolls or toys may help quiet an anxious child. Never perform any procedure on a young child without explaining it clearly in simple language. Use as few words as possible. Be positive and honest with the child. Do not provide too advanced a warning; otherwise, the child's fantasies may heighten his anxiety. Perform the procedure quickly after the explanation.

Geriatric Considerations

Elderly persons can experience considerable stress, but they do not react in the same way as younger persons. Severe anxiety is rare among the elderly. They do not seem to have the energy to fight or flee when stress occurs. Instead, they tend to accept, contemplate, and even show apathy as a means of coping.

Communicating with the Angry Client

In a health care setting a client may be angry over experiences with illness or over problems that existed before he sought health care. It is important for the nurse to understand that in many cases the client's ability to express anger is an essential part of his recovery.

Anger can represent rejection or disapproval of the nurse's care. The nurse should encourage the client to express anger openly and should not feel threatened by the client's words. When a client becomes angry, the nurse must not allow the emotion to compromise her care of him. The purpose of this skill is to assist the nurse in communicating with an angry client.

Potential Nursing Diagnoses

Impaired verbal communication related to feelings of anger
Ineffective individual coping related to anger
Dysfunctional grieving related to physical loss or chronic illness

Steps	Rationale
1. Physically prepare angry client and environment:	
■ Encourage other people, particularly those who provoke his anger, to leave room or area.	You want client to express his anger, but you do not want to provoke it.
■ Maintain adequate distance.	Avoids pressuring client. Also you should maintain a safe distance if anger becomes out of control.
■ Maintain an open exit.	Prevents feeling of being trapped.

Steps	Rationale
■ Make sure that your gestures are slow and deliberate rather than sudden and abrupt.	Less chance of misinterpretation of message and is less threatening.
■ Reduce disturbing factors in his room (e.g., noise, drafts, inadequate lighting).	Reduces irritating factors.
■ Take care of physical and emotional needs and discomforts.	Physical and emotional needs may be factors in client's anger. Sometimes he may not be aware of these needs.
2. Use physical attending:	
■ Begin with minimal intensity and very gradually increase.	Adequate personal space is very important with an angry client.
■ Begin with same type of position as client (when possible). Example: If client is standing, you stand. If client is sitting, you sit.	Conveys physically being "in tune" with another.
■ Gradually move to more relaxed position for both you and client. Example: If standing, eventually sit.	Facilitates less tense or less anxious exchange.
■ Keep your shoulders slightly down or relaxed.	Uses body language that is less intimidating or threatening.
■ Look toward client but avoid glaring or eye contact that is too intense.	Less intimidating.
■ Maintain "open" position. Avoid crossing your legs and arms. Keep hands unclenched and relaxed. Face slightly toward client.	Provides nonverbal cues of acceptance and listening that are congruent with attitude of acceptance.
3. Use psychological attending:	
■ Avoid defensive listening with an angry client.	In listening defensively instead of normally, you concentrate on your need to defend yourself or reasons why client should not feel angry.

Steps	Rationale
4. Introduce yourself and state who you are. Be brief and to the point.	Often client may not be able to listen or hear details of conversation. He may be concentrating only on his own point of view.
5. Respond to angry client: ■ Use therapeutic silence.	Often de-escalates anger, because anger expands emotional and physical energy and client runs out of momentum and energy to maintain anger at high level.
■ Use responses based on this hierarchy: description of experience, thoughts about experience, feelings that experience has generated.	Assists client in describing event causing anger and clarifying his thoughts and feelings.
■ Make vague statements more explicit or specific. Client: Nobody cares around here. Nurse: I'm not sure what you mean, Mr. Jones. Could you tell me more? Client: Everybody is just too busy. Nurse: What do you mean, everybody is just too busy? Client: I haven't seen anybody for 3 hours and I need my dressing changed before I go to physical therapy.	Angry client may have difficulty in being specific and needs assistance to do so. To change factors contributing to client's anger, you will often need specific information.
■ Practice accurate empathy.	This is ability to comprehend and communicate with accuracy thoughts, feelings, and experience of client in such a way that he would say, "Yes, that is exactly where I'm coming from." It is strong anger antidote.

Steps	Rationale
■ Explore alternatives to situation or feelings of anger.	May alter factors contributing to anger.
■ Present your perspective or point of view calmly and firmly.	May assist client to understand whole situation or another point of view. Also may assist in getting client to comply or follow through with care.
■ Use repeated assertion. Firmly repeat original response rather than argue each point.	Can be effective when client ignores, overreacts, or discounts your thoughts or feelings.
6. Use questions carefully:	
■ Make them open-ended and nonthreatening as much as possible.	Client becomes more willing to express himself.
■ Avoid numerous direct questions. Avoid using why and how.	Can intimidate and annoy client.
7. Don't let communication breakdown occur:	
■ Avoid attempts to show client why he should not be angry.	Client will react more to emotions than to reasoning.
■ Avoid aggressiveness or oversubmissive behavior.	Both tend to escalate client's anger.
■ Do not ignore client's anger.	You may lose opportunity to assist client in resolving anger.
■ Avoid trying to "out-talk" or give numerous explanations.	Annoys and irritates client.
8. Record in nurse's notes observations related to anger. Quote client exactly.	Aids in assessing source of client's anger.
■ Include nursing interventions in response to client's anger.	Documents your actions.

Nurse Alert

The nurse's failure to use proper techniques may increase a client's anger. It is important to remove factors contributing to anger (for example, do not ask a visitor to leave the room if the client desires company, cease any attempts to convince the client that he is wrong). Unless a potentially out-of-control situation is defused, the client may hurt himself or someone else.

Client Teaching

Teaching will be ineffective during a period when the client is angry, unless lack of knowledge is the source of his anger. Even then the nurse should limit explanations to simple discussions.

Pediatric Considerations

Anger is commonly expressed more frequently in individuals who are emotionally immature or impulsive (as in children).

Geriatric Considerations

The elderly client who suffers from an organic brain syndrome will often be impulsive and may become frustrated easily. Thus he also can become angry easily.

VITAL SIGNS

Measuring Oral Temperature

Normally a person's body temperature fluctuates within a relatively narrow range. Under control of the hypothalamus the body's core temperature stays within 0.6° of 37° C (1° of 98.6° F). Alterations may result from disease, infection, prolonged exposure to heat or cold, exercise, and hormonal disturbances. The body adapts to temperature changes by conserving or losing heat depending on the nature of the temperature alteration.

The oral method is the easiest way to obtain an accurate temperature reading. The nurse should delay measurement for 30 minutes if the client has ingested hot or cold liquids or food or has smoked. Each of these can cause false changes in temperature levels. During assessment of body temperature the nurse should consider the client's risks of temperature alterations. Conditions or therapies that can cause temperature alterations include expected or diagnosed infections, open wounds or burns, abnormal white cell count, use of immunosuppressive drugs, injury to the hypothalamus, lengthy exposure to temperature extremes, and reaction to blood products.

Potential Nursing Diagnoses

Fluid volume deficit related to diaphoresis
Hyperthermia related to infectious process

Equipment

Oral or stubby mercury-in-glass thermometer
Tissue paper
Disposable gloves

Steps	Rationale
1. Wash hands and apply disposable gloves.	Reduces transmission of microorganisms.
2. Hold tip of thermometer in your fingertips.	Prevents contamination of bulb to be inserted into client's mouth.
3. If thermometer is stored in a disinfectant solution, rinse it in cold water before using.	Removes potentially irritating disinfectant. Hot water might cause mercury to expand and break bulb.
4. Take soft tissue and wipe thermometer from bulb end toward fingers in a rotating manner. Dispose of tissue.	Rotating friction helps remove microorganisms. Wiping toward fingers prevents contamination of bulb end.
5. Read mercury level, holding thermometer at eye level. (Fig. 1)	Mercury is to be below 35.5° C (96° F). Thermometer reading must be below client's actual temperature before use.

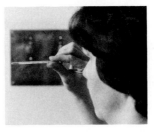

Fig. 1

6. If mercury is above desired level, shake thermometer down. Grasp tip of thermometer securely and stand away from any solid objects. Sharply flick wrist downward as though cracking a whip. Continue until reading is at appropriate level.	Brisk shaking lowers mercury level in glass tube. Standing in open spot prevents breakage of thermometer.

Steps	Rationale
7. Ask client to open his mouth and gently place thermometer in sublingual pocket (under tongue) lateral to center of lower jaw.	Heat from superficial blood vessels under the tongue produces temperature reading.
8. Ask client to hold thermometer with lips closed.	Maintains proper position of thermometer. Breakage of thermometer may injure oral mucosa and cause mercury poisoning.
9. Leave thermometer in place 2-3 minutes or according to agency policy.	Studies disagree as to proper length of time for recording. Graves and Markarian (1980) found that glass thermometers kept in place for 8 minutes recorded values on average only 0.07° F higher than those kept in for 3 minutes. Baker et. al (1984) found that 2-minute insertions did not cause clinically significant variations.
10. Carefully remove thermometer and read at eye level.	Gentle handling prevents client discomfort and ensures accurate reading.
11. Wipe off any secretions with a soft tissue. Wipe in rotating fashion from tip to bulb. Dispose of tissue.	Prevents contact of microorganisms with your hands. Tip is area of least contamination, bulb area of greatest contamination.
12. Wash thermometer in lukewarm soapy water. Rinse in cool water and dry.	Mechanically removes organic material that can hinder action of disinfectant.
13. Store thermometer in its container after shaking it down again.	Prevents breakage.

Steps	Rationale
14. Remove gloves, dispose of gloves, and wash hands.	Reduces transmission of micro-organisms.
15. Record client's temperature in proper chart or flow sheet.	Should be done immediately before it is forgotten.

Nurse Alert

Oral temperature measurement is contraindicated when the thermometer can injure the client or if the client is unable to hold the thermometer properly. Examples of contraindications include infants and small children, clients undergoing oral surgery or with pain in or trauma to the mouth, confused or unconscious clients, mouth breathers, clients with a history of convulsions, and clients with a shaking chill.

Client Teaching

Clients susceptible to temperature alterations should know how to measure their temperatures correctly so they can seek medical attention early when alterations occur. Parents of young children should learn to measure body temperature since children can develop seriously high fevers quickly.

Pediatric Considerations

Oral temperature measurement is not used in infants or small children. Most institutions recommend an age for permitting oral temperatures (for example, after 5 or 6 years). The immaturity of a child's temperature regulation mechanisms can cause sudden changes in body temperature. A newborn's body temperature normally ranges from 35.5° to 37.5° C (96° to 99.5° F).

Geriatric Considerations

Disturbances in temperature regulation that normally occur with aging can cause the elderly client to have a lower than normal body temperature.

Measuring Rectal Temperature

The nurse measures a client's body temperature rectally when use of an oral thermometer is contraindicated. The rectal site provides a reliable measure of body temperature. However, a client can easily become embarrassed when rectal temperature must be measured. Thus the nurse should take care to consider the client's privacy and comfort.

Certain conditions contraindicate rectal temperature measurement: a newborn infant, a client with rectal surgery or disorder, a client in pelvic or lower extremity traction or cast. Rectal temperature measurement is most reliable in young children.

Potential Nursing Diagnoses

Fluid volume deficit related to diaphoresis
Hyperthermia related to infectious process

Equipment

Rectal thermometer
Lubricant
Tissue paper
Disposable gloves

Steps	Rationale
1. Wash hands and don gloves.	Reduces transmission of micro-organisms.
2. Hold tip of thermometer in your fingertips.	This prevents contamination of the bulb to be inserted into client's rectum.

49

Steps	Rationale
3. If thermometer is stored in a disinfectant solution, rinse it in cold water before using.	Removes potentially irritating disinfectant. Hot water might cause mercury to expand and break bulb.
4. Wipe thermometer from bulb end toward fingers in a rotating manner. Dispose of tissue.	Rotating friction helps remove microorganisms. Wiping toward fingers prevents contamination of bulb end.
5. Read mercury level.	Mercury should be below 35.5° C (96° F) and below client's actual temperature before use.
6. If mercury is above desired level, shake thermometer down. Grasp upper end of thermometer securely and stand away from any solid objects. Sharply flick wrist downward as though cracking a whip. Continue until reading is at appropriate level.	Brisk shaking lowers mercury level in glass tube. Standing in an open spot away from objects prevents breakage of thermometer.
7. Draw curtains around client's bed or close room door. Keep client's upper body and lower extremities covered.	Maintains client privacy and minimizes embarrassment.
8. Assist client in assuming Sims' position, with upper leg flexed. Move aside bed linen to expose only anal area. Child may lie prone.	Provides optimal exposure of anal area for correct thermometer placement.
9. Squeeze liberal amount of water-soluble lubricant onto a tissue. Dip thermometer bulb end into lubricant, covering 2.5-3.5 cm (1-1½ inches) for adult or 1.2-2.5 cm (½-1 inch) for infant or child.	Inserting thermometer into lubricant container would contaminate all unused lubricant. Lubrication minimizes trauma to rectal mucosa during insertion.

Steps	Rationale
10. With nondominant hand raise client's upper buttock to expose anus.	Retracting buttocks fully exposes anus.
11. Gently insert thermometer into anus in direction of umbilicus. Insert 3.5 cm (1½ inches) for adult.	Proper insertion ensures adequate exposure to blood vessels in rectal wall.
12. Do not force thermometer. Ask client to take deep breath and blow out. Insert thermometer as client breathes deeply. If you feel resistance, withdraw thermometer immediately.	Gentle insertion prevents trauma to mucosa or breakage of thermometer. Taking deep breath helps to relax anal sphincter.
13. Hold thermometer in place 2-4 minutes according to agency policy. You may have to hold an infant's legs.	Holding thermometer prevents injury to client. Nichols and Kucha (1972) identified optimal placement time as 2 minutes.
14. Carefully remove thermometer.	Prevents injury to mucosa.
15. Wipe any secretions off with a tissue. Wipe down in a rotating fashion from tip to bulb. Dispose of tissue.	Prevents contacting microorganisms. Tip is area of least contamination, bulb area of greatest contamination.
16. Read thermometer.	
17. Wipe client's anal area to remove lubricant or feces.	Provides for client's comfort.
18. Help client return to a more comfortable position.	Restores client's comfort.
19. Wash thermometer in lukewarm soapy water and rinse in cool water.	Washing mechanically removes organic material that otherwise might be source of infection.
20. Dry thermometer and return it to its container after shaking it down.	Proper storage prevents breakage.

Steps	Rationale
21. Remove glove by pulling it off at wrist, turning it inside out. Discard gloves in proper receptacle.	Avoidance of contact with glove's outer surface minimizes spread of microorganisms
22. Wash your hands.	Reduces transmission of microorganisms.
23. Record client's temperature in proper chart or flow sheet. Signify rectal reading by capital *R*.	Vital signs should be recorded immediately after measurement. *R* prevents later confusion with oral or axillary measurements.

Nurse Alert

Always hold a rectal thermometer while it is in place. Sudden movement by the client could cause the thermometer to break in the rectum.

Client Teaching

Instruct mothers of young children how to position infant or small child. Infant or small child should be prone on the mother's lap or on a bed. The mother should gently retract both buttocks to expose the anus. The lubricated rectal thermometer is inserted 1.2 cm (½ inch) in an infant or small child.

Pediatric Considerations

Rectal temperature recording is contraindicated in newborns. Do not allow infants or young children to kick their legs or roll to the side while the thermometer is in place. The immaturity of a child's temperature regulation mechanisms can cause sudden changes in body temperature. A newborn's body temperature normally ranges between 35.5° and 37.5° C (96° and 99.5° F).

Geriatric Considerations

Disturbances in temperature regulation that normally occur with aging can cause elderly clients to have a lower than normal body temperature. An elderly person may have difficulty flexing his knee or hip to assume the Sims position. In that case, allow him to lie on his side with legs straight.

Measuring Axillary Temperature

The axillary temperature measurement is the safest method for assessing body temperature in a newborn. However, an axillary temperature is the least accurate of the three temperature measurement techniques because the thermometer must be placed against an external body site instead of an internal site. Whenever an oral or rectal thermometer can be safely used, the nurse should avoid using the axillary thermometer.

Potential Nursing Diagnoses

Fluid volume deficit related to diaphoresis
Hyperthermia related to infectious process

Equipment

Oral or stubby mercury-in-glass thermometer
Tissue paper

Steps	Rationale
1. Wash hands.	Reduces transmission of microorganisms.
2. Hold upper end of thermometer in your fingertips.	Prevents contamination of the bulb.
3. If thermometer is stored in disinfectant solution, rinse it in cold water before using.	Removes potentially irritating disinfectant. Hot water might cause mercury to expand and break bulb.
4. Wipe thermometer from bulb end toward finger in a rotating manner. Dispose of tissue.	Rotating friction helps remove microorganisms. Wiping toward fingers prevents contamination of bulb end.

53

Steps	Rationale
5. Read mercury level.	Mercury should be below 35.5° C (96° F) and below client's actual temperature before use.
6. If mercury is above desired level, shake thermometer down. Grasp upper end securely and stand away from any solid objects. Sharply flick wrist downward as though cracking a whip. Continue until reading is at appropriate level.	Brisk shaking lowers mercury level in glass tube. Standing in open spot prevents breakage of thermometer.
7. Draw curtains around bed and/or close room door.	Provides privacy and minimizes client embarrassment.
8. Assist client to a sitting or supine position.	Provides easy access to axilla.
9. Move clothing or gown away from client's shoulder and arm.	Provides optimal exposure of axilla.
10. Insert thermometer into center of client's axilla, lower arm over thermometer, and place forearm across his chest. (Fig. 2)	Maintains proper position of thermometer against blood vessels in axilla.

Fig. 2
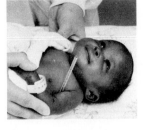

11. Hold thermometer in place for 5-10 minutes or according to agency policy.	Eoff and Joyce (1981) recommend 5 minutes for children. Recommended time varies among agencies.

Steps	Rationale
12. Remove thermometer and wipe off any secretions with tissue. Wipe in rotating fashion from fingers toward bulb. Dispose of tissue.	Avoids contact with microorganisms. Wipe from area of least contamination to area of most contamination.
13. Read thermometer.	Ensures accurate reading.
14. Wash thermometer in lukewarm soapy water. Rinse in cold water and dry.	Mechanically removes organic material that can interfere with disinfectant action.
15. Store thermometer in its container after shaking it down again.	Proper storage prevents breakage.
16. Assist client in replacing clothing or gown.	Restores client's sense of well-being.
17. Wash hands.	Reduces transmission of microorganisms.
18. Record temperature in proper chart or flow sheet. Signify axillary reading by capital *A*.	Vital signs should be recorded immediately after measurement. *A* prevents later confusion with oral or rectal measurements.

Nurse Alert

It may be necessary to gently hold the child's arm against his side.

Client Teaching

Instruct mothers of young children how to position and restrain the child properly. Also explain the importance of keeping the thermometer inserted at least 5 minutes (Eoff and Joyce, 1981).

Pediatric Considerations

Stay with the child throughout the procedure. The immaturity of a child's temperature regulation mechanisms can cause sudden changes in body temperature. A newborn's body temperature normally ranges between 35.5° and 37.5° C (96° and 99.5° F).

Geriatric Considerations

Disturbances in temperature regulation that normally occur with aging may cause the client to have a lower than normal body temperature.

Electronic Temperature

Measurement

Electronic thermometers are commonly used throughout various health care agencies. The device, consisting of a battery-powered display unit, thin wire cord, and temperature-sensitive probe, is capable of recording a client's body temperature in seconds. The electronic thermometer is not necessarily more accurate than a glass thermometer. The variables that alter temperature measurements (such as drinking hot or cold liquids) affect all types of thermometers. The advantages of the electronic thermometer are the quickness of recording and the safety from breakage and infection. Plastic probe covers protect clients when biting down during oral measurements and reduce cross-contamination between clients.

Potential Nursing Diagnoses

Hyperthermia related to infectious process

Equipment

Electronic thermometer with probe
Probe cover
Lubricant (for rectal measurement)
Disposable gloves

Steps	Rationale
1. Wash hands.	Reduces transmission of micro-organisms.
2. Close room door or bedside curtain.	Provides for client privacy.
3. Assist client to appropriate position for access to selected temperature site.	Ensures correct thermometer placement and accurate readings.

Steps	Rationale
4. Choose correct temperature probe (usually color coded blue for oral or axillary and red for rectal) and connect to electronic display unit. (Fig. 3)	Separate probes prevent contamination of body cavities during use.

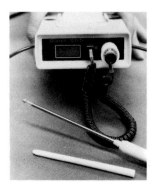

Fig. 3

Steps	Rationale
5. Make sure that display window shows no temperature reading.	Will ensure proper registering of client's temperature.
6. Grasp probe at top, without pushing ejection button.	Ejection button ejects probe cover.
7. Place clean disposable plastic cover over temperature probe.	Prevents transmission of microorganisms between clients.
8. Explain procedure to client.	Certain clients may be unfamiliar with measuring device. Explanation will relieve client anxiety.
9. Apply disposable gloves.	Reduces transmission of blood-borne pathogens. Gloves should be worn when handling items soiled by body fluids (CDC, 1987).
10. Insert probe into selected body site, following same techniques as with mercury thermometers.	Ensures accurate readings. Correct techniques prevent injury to client.

Steps	Rationale
11. Keep probe in place until electronic unit alarms and temperature reading appears on digital display.	Electronic units are capable of registering client's body temperature in seconds.
12. Note temperature reading.	
13. Gently remove probe and eject probe cover into trash receptacle by pushing ejection button.	Reduces spread of infection.
14. Replace probe in electronic unit.	Battery unit is rechargeable.
15. Help client return to desired comfortable position.	Maintains client's sense of well-being.
16. Wash your hands and dispose of gloves.	Reduces transmission of microorganisms.
17. Record temperature in vital signs flow sheet or nurse's notes.	Vital signs should be recorded immediately for accuracy.

Nurse Alert

Use whatever precautions are necessary to restrain the client or to hold the probe in place without injuring the client.

Client Teaching

Electronic thermometers are rarely used in the home setting. Thus explanation of the procedure is all that is necessary.

Pediatric Considerations

Carefully restrain a child to prevent the probe from injuring the oral or rectal tissues. Risk of injury is less than with glass thermometers. (Refer to previous temperature measurement skills.)

Geriatric Considerations

For rectal measurements, an elderly client may require assistance with positioning due to musculoskeletal disabilities. Remember, an elderly person's body temperature can normally be lower than that of a younger adult.

Assessing Radial Pulse

The character of a client's pulse provides valuable data regarding the integrity of his cardiovascular system.

The nurse commonly assesses the radial artery pulse during routine measurement of a client's vital signs or when a change is expected in his condition. The radial pulse is usually the most accessible. When it is inaccessible because of a dressing, cast, or other encumbrance, the apical pulse can be assessed instead. This involves auscultating heart sounds with a stethoscope placed medially below the left nipple (Skill 2-6).

Before assessing a client's pulse, the nurse attempts to control four factors—exercise, anxiety, pain, and postural change—that might cause false elevations or drops in heart rate. The nurse should also be able to anticipate how certain medications or disease processes will affect the client's heart rate.

Potential Nursing Diagnoses

Decreased cardiac output related to conduction or contractility deficit

Altered peripheral tissue perfusion related to arterial obstruction

Potential activity intolerance related to impaired cardiac output

Equipment

Wristwatch with second hand or digital display

Steps	Rationale
1. Wash hands.	Reduces chances of transmitting microorganisms.
2. Explain purpose and method of procedure to client.	Relieves client anxiety and facilitates his cooperation during procedure.

Steps	Rationale
3. Have client assume a supine or sitting position. If supine, place his arm across his lower chest with wrist extended and palm down. If sitting, bend his elbow 90 degrees and support his lower arm on chair or on your arm. Extend his wrist with palm down.	Proper positioning fully exposes radial artery for palpation.
4. Place tips of first two fingers of your hand over groove along radial or thumb side of client's inner wrist. (Fig. 4)	Fingertips are most sensitive parts of hand to palpate arterial pulsations. Nurse's thumb has pulsation that may interfere with accuracy.

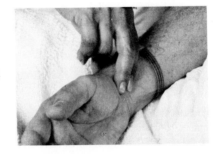

Fig. 4

5. Lightly compress against radius, obliterate pulse initially, and then relax pressure so pulse becomes easily palpable.	Pulse is more accurately assessed with moderate pressure. Too much pressure occludes pulse and impairs blood flow.
6. When pulse can be felt regularly, use watch's second hand and begin to count rate, starting with zero, and then one, etc.	Rate is determined accurately only after assessor is assured that pulse can be palpated. Timing should begin with zero. Count of 1 is first beat felt after timing begins.
7. If pulse is regular, count for 15 seconds and multiply total by 4.	Regular rate can be accurately assessed in 15 seconds.

Steps	Rationale
8. If pulse is irregular, count for full minute.	Ensures accurate count.
9. Assess regularity and frequency of any existing dysrhythmia.	Inefficient contraction of heart fails to transmit pulse wave and can interfere with cardiac output.
10. Determine strength of pulse. Note thrust of pulse against fingertips.	Strength reflects volume of blood ejected against arterial wall with each heart contraction.
11. Assist client to comfortable position.	Promotes sense of well-being.
12. Record characteristics of pulse in medical record or flow sheet. Report abnormalities to nurse in charge or physician.	Provides data for monitoring changes in client's condition. Abnormalities may necessitate medical therapy.
13. Wash hands.	Reduces transmission of microorganisms.

Nurse Alert

If the nurse detects an irregular rhythm, it is important to assess for a pulse deficit. Compare the pulses at the radial artery and the apex of the heart. A difference between rates indicates a deficit.

Client Teaching

Certain clients should learn how to assess their own pulse. Those receiving medications that affect heart function should assess their pulse as well as any undesirable effects of medications. Clients undergoing cardiovascular and pulmonary rehabilitation should also assess their pulse to determine exercise tolerance.

Pediatric Considerations

A 1-week-old to 3-month-old infant's resting heart rate ranges from 110 to 220 beats per minute. By the age of 2 years, child's resting heart rate ranges from 80 to 150 beats per minute. From the ages of 2 to 10 years the rate ranges from 70 to 110. By the time the child is 10 years of age the resting heart ranges from 55 to 90 beats per minute.

Geriatric Considerations

In the healthy older adult the resting heart rate should range between 60 to 100 beats per minute. Older adults with cardiovascular, pulmonary, or other chronic illnesses are at risk for rapid, slow, or irregular heart rate and rhythms.

Assessing Apical
Pulse

The apical pulse is assessed with a stethoscope. The stethoscope is placed over the apex of the client's heart. The stethoscope enables the sounds originating from the valves of the heart to be transmitted via the rubber tubing to the nurse's ears for pulse assessment.

The apical pulse is the best site for assessing an infant's or young child's pulse. When a client takes medication that affects heart rate, the apical pulse may provide a more accurate assessment of cardiac rate and rhythm.

Potential Nursing Diagnoses

Decreased cardiac output related to irregular pulse
Activity intolerance related to irregular pulse
Anxiety related to irregular pulse

Equipment

Stethoscope
Wristwatch with second hand or digital display

Steps	Rationale
1. Clean earpieces and diaphragm of stethoscope with alcohol swab as needed.	Controls transmission of microorganisms when nurses share stethoscope.
2. Wash hands.	Reduces transmission of microorganisms.
3. Close door or draw curtains around client's bed.	Maintains client's privacy.

Steps	Rationale
4. With client in supine or sitting position, turn down bed linen and raise gown, or remove client's upper garments to expose sternum and left side of chest.	Exposes portion of chest wall for selection of auscultatory site.
5. Palpate angle of Louis, located just below suprasternal notch at point where horizontal ridge is felt along body of sternum. Place index finger just to the left of client's sternum and palpate second intercostal space below and proceed downward until fifth intercostal space is palpated. Move index finger horizontally along fifth intercostal space to left midclavicular line (Fig. 5). Palpate point of maximal impulse (PMI), also called Erb's point.	Use of anatomical landmarks allows the nurse to place stethoscope over apex of heart. This position enhances ability to hear heart sounds clearly. The PMI is over the apex of the heart.

Fig. 5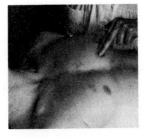

6. Place diaphragm of stethoscope in palm of your hand for 5-10 seconds.	Warms diaphragm and reduces risk of client being startled.

Steps	Rationale
7. Place diaphragm over PMI and auscultate for normal S_1 and S_2 (lub, dub) heart sounds. (Fig. 6)	Heart sounds are the result of blood moving through cardiac valves.

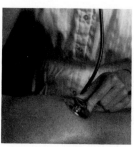

Fig. 6

Steps	Rationale
8. If S_1 and S_2 sounds are heard with regularity, use watch secondhand and count for 30 seconds and multiply by 2.	Rate is determined accurately only after nurse is able to auscultate sounds clearly.
9. If heart rate is irregular, count for 60 seconds.	Rate determined is more accurate when measured over a longer interval.
10. Replace client's garments and bed linen.	Maintains client comfort and privacy.
11. Wash hands.	Reduces transmission of microorganisms.
12. Record characteristics of pulse on flow sheet. Report any abnormalities to nurse in charge or client's physician.	Provides data for monitoring changes in client's condition. Abnormalities may require medical therapy.

Nurse Alert

The nurse should note the presence of any irregularity. If this ir-regularity is new to the client, it should be reported to the nurse in charge or the client's physician. In addition, irregularities can be associated with adverse effects of cardiac medications, e.g., digoxin.

Client Teaching

Family members may need to learn to take the client's apical pulse in the home setting. The nurse needs to teach the caregiver how to correctly use the stethoscope as well as how to correctly obtain an apical pulse.

Pediatric Considerations

In infants and small children the most accurate site for pulse as-sessment is the apical site.

Geriatric Considerations

The healthy older adult has a normal cardiac rate and rhythm. However, in the presence of cardiac medications or chronic ill-nesses the nurse should assess the pulse apically.

Assessing
Respirations

When the nurse assesses a client's respirations, the procedure involves observing the rate, depth, and rhythm of his ventilatory movements. The nurse must be able to recognize normal passive breathing compared with ventilations that require muscular effort. Minimal effort is required to inhale and even less to exhale. If a client is having respiratory difficulties, the intercostal and accessory muscles will work more actively and the nurse will be able to see pronounced movement of his shoulder, neck, and chest muscles.

The nurse should be familiar with factors that normally affect respirations as well as conditions that place a client at risk of respiratory alterations.

Potential Nursing Diagnoses

Ineffective airway clearance related to pain, position restrictions, or fatigue

Ineffective breathing pattern related to effects of analgesics, pain, or pulmonary infection

Equipment

Wristwatch with second hand or digital display

Steps	Rationale
1. Be sure that client is in comfortable position, preferably sitting.	Discomfort can cause client to breathe more rapidly.

Steps	Rationale
2. Place client's arm in relaxed position across his abdomen or lower chest, or place your hand directly over client's upper abdomen.	This position is used during assessment of pulse. Both your and the client's hands rise and fall during respiratory cycle. Measuring respirations immediately after pulse assessment makes measurement inconspicuous.
3. Observe complete respiratory cycle (one inspiration and one expiration).	Ensures that count will begin with normal respiratory cycle.
4. Once a cycle is observed, look at watch's second hand and begin to count rate: when second hand hits number on dial, count "one" to begin first full cycle.	Timing begins with count of one. Respirations occur more slowly than pulse; thus count begins with one.
5. For an adult, count number of respirations in 30 seconds and multiply by 2. For infant or young child, count respirations for full minute.	Respiratory rate is equivalent to number of respirations per minute. Young infants and children breathe in an irregular rhythm.
6. If an adult's respirations have irregular rhythm or are abnormally slow or fast, count for full minute.	Accurate interpretation requires assessment for at least 1 minute.
7. While counting, note whether depth is shallow, normal, or deep and whether rhythm is normal or contains altered patterns.	The character of ventilatory movements may reveal specific alterations or disease states.
8. Record results in chart or flow sheet. Report any signs of respiratory alterations.	Provides data for monitoring change in client's condition. Abnormalities may indicate need for therapy.

Nurse Alert

Clients' respiratory patterns can change for a variety of reasons. Some reasons, such as an asthmatic attack or the presence of foreign body airway obstruction, are more critical than others and require rapid interventions. In addition, pain and anxiety can also alter respiratory patterns. The nurse should not dismiss changes in respiration without further assessment.

Client Teaching

Clients with chronic lung disease can benefit from diaphragmatic breathing exercises (see Skill 12-1).

Pediatric Considerations

The nurse should plan on assessing respirations as the first vital sign in an infant or child. Startling or arousing an infant for other preliminary measurements can falsely increase respirations. Usually the nurse can simply observe respirations as the infant or young child lies in bed with his chest and abdomen uncovered.

A newborn breathes at a rate of 30 to 60 respirations per minute. A 2-year-old breathes 20 to 30 respirations per minute. A 6-year-old has a rate of 18 to 26 breaths per minute.

Geriatric Considerations

An adult normally breathes 12 to 20 respirations per minute at rest. With advancing age the average respiratory rate increases and chest expansion tends to decline due to increased rigidity of the chest wall.

Assessing Blood Pressure
by Auscultation

For blood to flow throughout the circulatory system the heart pumps it into the arteries under high pressure. Pressure within the aorta at the time of left ventricular contraction (systole) is approximately 120 mm Hg in a healthy adult who is upright but not exercising. Once the aorta distends, a pressure wave traveling through the arterial system sends blood to the peripheral tissues. As the ventricles relax, pressure in the arterial system falls. The diastolic pressure (normally 80 mm Hg) is the minimal pressure exerted against the arterial walls. The nurse records blood pressure with the systolic before the diastolic reading (for example, 120/80).

The nurse's assessment of blood pressure helps determine the balance of several hemodynamic factors: cardiac output, peripheral vascular resistance, blood volume and viscosity, elasticity of the arteries. A client's blood pressure should be carefully compared with pulse rate and character in addition to other cardiovascular assessment findings so an intelligent conclusion can be drawn regarding the client's circulatory status.

Potential Nursing Diagnoses

Decreased cardiac output related to hypovolemia
Altered cardiopulmonary and peripheral tissue perfusion related to hypovolemia

Equipment

Stethoscope
Sphygmomanometer with cuff

Steps	Rationale
1. Determine proper cuff size. Width of inflatable bladder within cuff should be 40% of circumference at midpoint of limb on which cuff is to be used (or 20% wider than diameter). Length of bladder should be about twice recommended width.	Proper cuff size is necessary so correct amount of pressure is applied over artery. Cuffs that are too narrow, too wide, or improperly applied cause false-high or false-low readings, respectively.
2. Determine best site for cuff placement. Avoid extremity with an IV, arteriovenous shunt, presence of trauma.	Application of pressure from an inflated cuff can temporarily impair blood flow and compromise circulation.
3. Explain to client purpose of procedure.	Reassures client.
4. Wash hands.	Reduces transmission of microorganisms.
5. Assist client to comfortable sitting position, with arm slightly flexed, forearm supported at heart level, and palm turned up.	Having arm above level of heart produces false-low readings. This position facilitates cuff application.
6. Expose client's upper arm fully.	Ensures proper cuff application.

Steps	Rationale
7. Palpate brachial artery (on lower medial side of biceps muscle). Position cuff 2.5 cm (1 inch) above site of pulsations (antecubital fossa). (Fig. 7)	Stethoscope will be placed over artery without touching cuff.

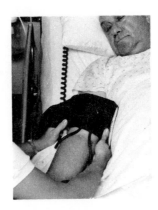

Fig. 7

8. Center arrows marked on cuff along brachial artery.	Inflating bladder directly over brachial artery ensures that proper pressure is applied during inflation.
9. With cuff fully deflated, wrap cuff evenly and snugly around upper arm.	Loose-fitting cuff causes false elevations in blood pressure readings.
10. Be sure that manometer is positioned at eye level.	Ensures accurate reading of mercury level.
11. Place stethoscope earpieces in your ears and be sure sounds are clear, not muffled.	Each earpiece should follow angle of your ear canal to facilitate hearing.

Steps	Rationale
12. Relocate brachial artery and place diaphragm (or bell) of stethoscope over it. (Fig. 8)	Ensures optimal sound reception. American Heart Association recommends use of bell for detecting low-pitched Korotkoff sounds.

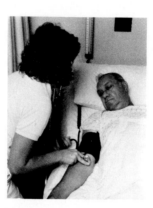

Fig. 8

Steps	Rationale
13. Close valve of pressure bulb clockwise until tight.	Prevents air leak during inflation.
14. Inflate cuff to 30 mm Hg above client's normal systolic level.	Ensures accurate pressure measurement.
15. Slowly release valve, allowing mercury to fall at rate of 2-3 mm Hg per second.	Too rapid or too slow decline in mercury level may lead to inaccurate reading.
16. Note point on manometer at which first clear sound is heard.	First Korotkoff sound indicates systolic pressure.
17. Continue to deflate cuff gradually, noting point at which sound becomes muffled or dampened.	Fourth Korotkoff sound may be detected as diastolic pressure in adults with hypertension. American Heart Association recommends it as indication of diastolic pressure in children.

Steps	Rationale
18. Continue cuff deflation and note point at which sound disappears.	American Heart Association recommends recording fifth Korotkoff sound as diastolic pressure in adults.
19. Deflate cuff rapidly and remove it from client's arm unless you need to repeat measurement.	Continuous inflation causes arterial occlusion, resulting in numbness and tingling (paresthesia) of client's arm.
20. If repeating procedure, wait 30 seconds.	Prevents venous congestion and falsely high readings.
21. Fold cuff and store it properly.	Proper maintenance of supplies contributes to instrument accuracy.
22. Assist client to position he prefers and cover his upper arm.	Maintains client's comfort.
23. Record findings on medical record or flow sheet.	Should be done immediately.
24. Wash hands.	Reduces transmission of microorganisms.

Nurse Alert

Be aware of signs and symptoms of high blood pressure (hypertension): headache (usually occipital), flushing of the face, nosebleed, fatigue in elderly clients. Be aware also of the signs and symptoms of low blood pressure (hypotension): dizziness, mental confusion, restlessness, pale or cyanotic (dusky) skin and mucous membranes, cool mottled skin over the extremities.

Client Teaching

Clients should understand the risk factors of high blood pressure: obesity, increased sodium intake, increased cholesterol intake, smoking, lack of exercise. When clients are taking antihypertensive medications, review their medication schedules and assess their understanding of the purpose and importance of the medication.

Pediatric Considerations

A newborn (3000 g or 6.6 pounds) has an average systolic pressure of 50 to 52, diastolic of 25 to 30, and mean of 35 to 40 mm Hg. At 4 years the average blood pressure is 85/60; at 6 years it averages 95/62; and at 12 years, 108/67.

Geriatric Considerations

With aging there is a reduction in blood vessel compliance and an increase in peripheral resistance to blood flow. Arteriosclerosis is a common disorder with advancing age, although it can begin early in adulthood. Because of vascular changes, elderly clients are at risk of significantly increased systolic and slightly increased diastolic pressures.

POSITIONING
AND
TRANSFER

Proper Lifting

The nurse is at risk for injury to lumbar muscles in lifting, transferring, or positioning the partly or totally immobilized client. Injury to the lumbar area affects the ability to bend forward, backward, and side to side. In addition, the ability to rotate the hips and lower back is decreased.

As more clients are being discharged into the home setting for continuing care, it is necessary for the nurse to teach members of the client's family to safely lift and transfer the client.

The purpose of this skill and all skills in this unit is to teach both the nurse and family members how to safely and correctly lift and transfer the client with impaired mobility.

Potential Nursing Diagnoses

Impaired skin integrity related to decreased mobility
Bathing/hygiene self-care deficit related to decreased mobility
Potential for injury related to improper lifting

Steps	Rationale
1. Assess "basic four" lifting measures: position of object, height of object, body position, and maximum weight.	Determines need for assistance from additional personnel during lift.
2. Come close to object to be moved.	Increases your body balance during lift.
3. Enlarge your base of support, placing feet apart.	Maintains better body balance, reducing your risk of falling.

Steps	Rationale
4. Lower your center of gravity to object to be lifted. Flex at knees and hips. (Fig. 9)	Increases body balance and enables your muscle groups to work together in synchronized manner.

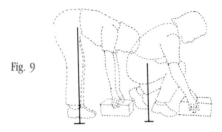

Fig. 9

Steps	Rationale
5. Maintain proper alignment of head and neck with vertebrae.	Reduces risk of injuring your lumbar vertebrae and muscle groups.

Nurse Alert

Before lifting an object, the nurse should decide if she will be able to safely lift it alone. If she feels that she cannot (the object is too large or too heavy), she should seek additional personnel to help her.

Client Teaching

Demonstrating correct lifting techniques is an excellent way for the nurse to teach the client and family how they can avoid injuring themselves when moving something.

Geriatric Considerations

The geriatric client may require re-education on what he can and cannot safely lift. Objects that could be safely lifted in the middle and late adult years cannot usually be lifted in the later adult years.

Ensuring Proper Positioning

Correct positioning of a client is crucial for maintaining proper body alignment. Any client with impaired mobility is at risk of developing contractures, postural abnormalities, and pressure sores. The nurse has the primary responsibility to minimize this risk, which is done by changing the position of the client having impaired mobility and decreased sensation at frequent intervals.

Potential Nursing Diagnoses

Impaired physical mobility related to fatigue
Impaired skin integrity related to immobility
Altered peripheral tissue perfusion related to immobility

Steps	Rationale
1. Wash hands.	Reduces transmission of micro-organisms.
2. Determine what equipment is needed. Organize work area. Remove obstacles.	Provides for safe, organized positioning.
3. Tell client what you are doing and what he can do to help.	Enables you to use client's mobility and strength, if possible.
4. Determine if you will need assistance and get it before beginning to change client's position.	Gives you an opportunity to assess your ability to move client independently and ensures your safety as well as that of client.
5. Elevate the bed to a comfortable height.	Elevates the level of work toward the nurse's center of gravity.

Steps	Rationale
6. Place one pillow beneath client's head.	Provides support to head without causing flexion, hyperextension, or lateral flexion of neck.
7. Determine that client's elbows, knees, and hips are supported and slightly flexed.	Ensures proper alignment when these joints are supported. Flexion prevents prolonged hyperextension, which could impair joint mobility.
8. Determine that client's feet are supported. If he is in bed, provide footboard or sandbags, if necessary. If in chair or wheelchair, position his feet flat on floor, on footrest of wheelchair, or on another support device.	Support maintains dorsal flexion and helps prevent footdrop.
9. Determine that his extremities are supported and, whenever possible, in positions for free movement.	Reduces risk of joint dislocation, particularly when there is underlying nerve damage (as after stroke). Allowing extremity to move freely helps maintain joint mobility.
10. Check that any bony prominences are not permitted to remain in direct contact with other parts of his body (e.g., knee resting on thigh of other leg in side-lying position).	Pressure increases risk of skin breakdown and damage to musculoskeletal system.
11. Change his body position at least every 2 hours.	Removes pressure from dependent body tissues, lessening risk of venous pooling.
12. Wash your hands.	Reduces transmission of microorganisms.
13. Record in nurse's notes status of client's skin and underlying tissue and client's new position.	Documents the current integrity of the client's skin and which positioning procedure was performed.

Nurse Alert

When positioning clients, the nurse must be aware of the fact that certain traumatic or postoperative conditions require the client to be placed in specific positions. For example, a supine position may be necessary for clients after some spinal surgery.

Client Teaching

Teach the client which position or positions are appropriate to decrease stress on the musculoskeletal system. Inform the client regarding the hazards of immobilization and the early signs of skin breakdown and impaired joint mobility. Assist the client in relaxation techniques.

Pediatric Considerations

The pediatric client usually requires positioning to maintain alignment of a fractured extremity or to prevent accidental removal of a tube or drain. Nursing measures must be designed to safely restrain the young child as well as prevent him from changing positions.

Geriatric Considerations

An elderly client is at greater risk than a younger client of skin breakdown or joint deformities related to immobility. Therefore his nursing care plan may require more frequent position changes, such as every hour or every 90 minutes instead of every 2 hours.

Supported Fowler
Position

The supported Fowler position improves cardiac output and ventilation as well as facilitates urinary and bowel elimination. In this position the head of the client's bed is raised 45 to 60 degrees and the client's knees are slightly elevated so there will be no restriction of circulation to the lower extremities. Proper alignment of the body when the client is in this position requires support that maintains comfort and reduces the risk of damage to body systems.

Potential Nursing Diagnoses

Impaired skin integrity related to immobility
Altered peripheral tissue perfusion related to immobility
Ineffective breathing patterns related to immobility

Steps	Rationale
1. Wash hands.	Reduces transmission of micro-organisms.
2. Position client supine with his head near headboard.	Prevents client from sliding toward foot of bed when head of bed is elevated.
3. Raise head of bed 45-60 degrees.	Increases client comfort, improves breathing, and increases his opportunity to socialize, relax, or watch television.
4. Allow client's head to rest against mattress or on very small pillow.	Prevents flexion contracture of client's cervical vertebrae.

Steps	Rationale
5. If large pillow is used, turn it lengthwise to support client's upper back, shoulders, and head.	Prevents flexion contracture of his cervical vertebrae and maintains vertebral alignment.
6. Use pillows to support client's arms and hands if he does not have voluntary control or use of upper extremities.	Prevents shoulder dislocation from downward gravitational pull of unsupported arms, promotes circulation by preventing venous pooling, reduces edema in hands or arms, and prevents flexion contractures of wrist.
7. Position pillow at client's lower back.	Supports lumbar vertebrae and decreases spinal flexion.
8. Place small pillow or roll under client's thighs. If his lower extremities are paraiyzed or he is unable to control lower extremities, use a roll under his trochanters in addition to a pillow under his thighs. (Fig. 10)	Prevents hyperextension of knees and occlusion of popliteal artery due to pressure from body weight. Trochanter roll prevents external rotation of legs.

Fig. 10

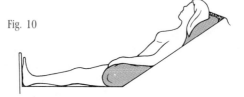

| 9. Place small pillow or roll under client's ankle region. | Eliminates prolonged pressure from bed on heels. |

Steps	Rationale
10. Place footboard (Fig. 10) or foot-drop stops (Fig. 11) at bottom of client's feet.	Maintains feet in dorsiflexion. Reduces risk of foot-drop.

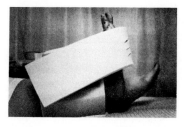

Fig. 11

Steps	Rationale
11. Wash your hands.	Reduces transmission of micro-organisms.
12. Record in nurse's notes client's new position.	Documents that procedure was performed.

Nurse Alert

Clients in the Fowler position are at risk of cervical flexion contractures if the pillow is too thick. Additional complications may include external rotation of the hips, foot-drop, and skin breakdown at the sacrum and heels.

Client Teaching

The Fowler position provides an excellent opportunity for the nurse to implement client teaching in self-care (as with the newly diagnosed diabetic client), skin care, and knowledge about medications.

Geriatric Considerations

Elderly clients are at greater risk than younger clients of skin breakdown due to increased capillary fragility, decreased muscle mass, and reduced skin moisture.

Supported Supine Position

The supine position, also called the dorsal recumbent position, may be required after spinal surgery and the administration of some spinal anesthetics. In this position the relationship of body parts is essentially the same as in proper standing alignment except that the body is horizontal.

Potential Nursing Diagnoses

Impaired skin integrity related to immobility
Altered peripheral tissue perfusion related to immobility

Steps	Rationale
1. Wash hands.	Reduces transmission of micro-organisms.
2. Place client flat in center of bed.	Prepares client for proper positioning.
3. Place pillow under client's shoulders, neck, and head, unless contraindicated following some spinal surgery or anesthetic administration.	Maintains correct alignment and prevents flexion contracture as well as hyperextension of cervical vertebrae.

Steps	Rationale
4. Place small pillow or roll under client's lumbar spine. (Fig. 12)	Provides support to lumbar vertebrae, especially when firm mattress is being used, and reduces flexion of lumbar vertebrae.

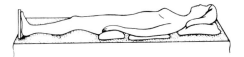

Fig. 12

Steps	Rationale
5. When necessary, place rolls under client's trochanters or sandbags parallel with lateral surface of his thighs.	Reduces external rotation of the legs.
6. Place small pillow or roll under his upper legs to flex knees slightly.	Prevents hyperextension of knees and improves circulation by reducing pressure from bed on the popliteal artery.
7. Place small pillow or roll under client's ankles to elevate heels.	Raising heels from surface of bed reduces pressure on them.
8. Place footboard or foot-drop stops against bottom of client's feet.	Maintains feet in dorsiflexion. Reduces risk of foot-drop.
9. Place pillows under client's forearms, maintaining upper arms parallel with his body. (Fig. 13)	Reduces internal rotation of shoulders and prevents extension of elbows.

Fig. 13

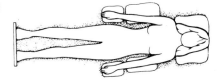

Steps	Rationale
10. Have client grasp hand rolls or towels or use hand splints when available.	Reduces extension of fingers and abduction of thumb. Also maintains thumb slightly adducted and in opposition to the fingers.
11. Wash your hands.	Reduces transmission of microorganisms.
12. Record in nurse's notes client's new position.	Documents that procedure was performed.

Nurse Alert

Clients in the supine position are at risk of internal rotation of the shoulders, external rotation of the hips, foot-drop, and pressure sores at the lumbar vertebrae, elbows, heels, and scapulas.

Client Teaching

While the client is supine, the nurse can teach him and his family the prescribed range of joint motion exercises and skin care measures.

Pediatric Considerations

A child may be restrained in the supine position to maintain patency of an intravenous catheter or the integrity of postoperative drains. The nurse should incorporate into her plan of care time to hold and play with the child.

Geriatric Considerations

Elderly clients are at greater risk than younger clients of skin breakdown due to increased capillary fragility, decreased muscle mass, and reduced skin moisture.

Supported Prone Position

The primary therapeutic use of the prone position is to provide an alternative for clients who are immobilized or on prolonged bedrest. It is not a well-tolerated position, and frequent changes are required to relieve boredom and discomfort.

Potential Nursing Diagnoses

Impaired skin integrity related to immobility
Potential for injury related to risk of aspiration

Steps	Rationale
1. Wash hands.	Reduces transmission of micro-organisms.
2. Place client on his abdomen in center of bed.	Prepares client for proper positioning.
3. Turn client's head to one side and support with small pillow. When excessive drainage from mouth is present, pillow may be contraindicated. (Fig. 14)	Reduces flexion or hyperextension of cervical vertebrae.

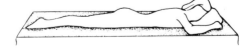

Fig. 14

Steps	Rationale
4. Place small pillow under client's belly below level of diaphragm.	Reduces pressure on breasts in some female clients, decreases hyperextension of lumbar vertebrae, and improves breathing by reducing pressure on diaphragm from mattress.
5. Position client toward foot of bed so his feet hang over mattress, or support lower legs with pillow to elevate toes. (Fig. 15)	Prevents foot-drop and reduces external rotation of legs and pressure on toes from mattress.

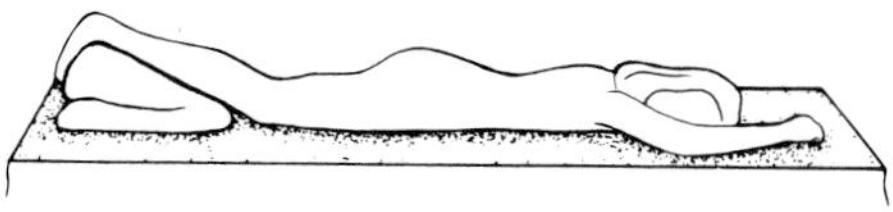

Fig. 15

6. Wash your hands.	Reduces transmission of micro-organisms.
7. Record in nurse's notes client's new position.	Documents that procedure was performed.

Nurse Alert

When placing a client in the prone position, the nurse should be sure that a pillow is under the client's lower legs to promote dorsiflexion of the ankles and knee flexion. Body alignment is poor when the ankles are continuously in plantar flexion and the lumbar spine remains hyperextended. In addition, the nurse must frequently assess the client's breathing patterns to detect any alterations that might result from the prone position.

Client Teaching

When the client is prone, the nurse can effectively teach his family about skin care or any dressing changes on the back that may be required.

Pediatric Considerations

Children placed prone usually do not tolerate the position well because of limited eye contact with their environment. When the prone position is required, the nurse should incorporate quiet play or stories into her plan of care.

Geriatric Considerations

Elderly clients may become disoriented when in the prone position because of decreased visual cues from their environment. The nurse can reduce this risk by placing a clock within the client's visual field, increasing the amount of time she spends with the client, and encouraging visitation by family.

Supported Side-Lying (Lateral) Position

The side-lying position removes pressure from any bony prominences on the client's back and redistributes the major portion of his body weight on the dependent hip and shoulder. In this position the client's trunk alignment should be the same as in proper standing posture.

Potential Nursing Diagnoses

Impaired skin integrity related to immobility
Altered peripheral tissue perfusion related to immobility

Steps	Rationale
1. Wash hands.	Reduces transmission of microorganisms.
2. Place client supine in center of bed.	Aligns client properly.
3. Roll client onto his side.	Prepares him for proper positioning.
4. Place pillow under client's head and neck.	Maintains alignment, reduces lateral flexion of neck, and decreases muscle strain on major neck muscle (sternocleidomastoid).
5. Both his arms should be slightly flexed: upper arm supported by a pillow under the forearm, lower arm supported by the mattress.	Decreases internal rotation and adduction of shoulder, preventing dislocation. Supporting both arms in a slightly flexed position protects joints and improves ventilation because chest is able to expand more easily.

Steps	Rationale
6. Place one or two pillows under client's upper leg. Pillows should support leg evenly from groin to foot. (Fig. 16)	Prevents internal rotation and adduction of thigh and reduces pressure to bony prominences of leg from mattress.

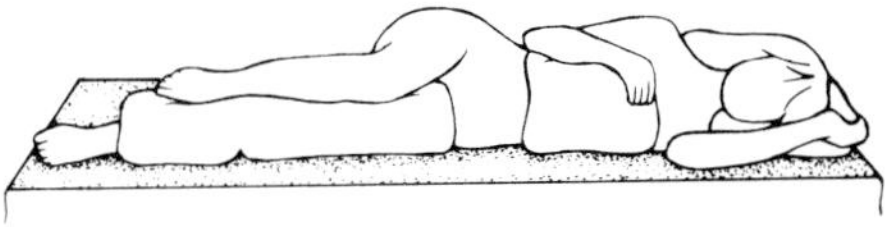

Fig. 16

7. Place supports, such as sandbags or foot-drop stops, at client's feet.	Maintains feet in dorsiflexion. Reduces risk of foot-drop.
8. Place rolled pillow parallel with client's back.	Maintains support and alignment of vertebrae. Also keeps client from rolling back out of alignment and prevents rotation of spine.
9. Wash your hands.	Reduces transmission of microorganisms.
10. Record in nurse's notes client's new position.	Documents that procedure was performed.

Nurse Alert

When placing a client in the side-lying position, the nurse should use caution to avoid lateral flexion of the neck, improper spinal alignment, internal rotation of the hips and shoulder joints, footdrop, and pressure on the ilium, knees, and ankles.

Client Teaching

The side-lying position provides the nurse an excellent opportunity to teach the client (and family) about therapeutic measures that may be continued in the home.

Pediatric Considerations

The side-lying position is used with an unconscious, immobilized, or burned child. If the child is alert, the nurse should incorporate quiet diversional activities into her care plan so this position will be maintained.

Geriatric Considerations

Elderly clients are at greater risk than younger clients of skin breakdown caused by increased capillary fragility, decreased muscle mass, and reduced skin moisture.

Supported Sims
(Semiprone) Position

The Sims position is frequently used for an unconscious client to increase drainage of mucus from the mouth. In addition, it provides an alternative for clients who are immobilized or on bedrest. In this position the client's weight is placed on the anterior ilium and the humerus and clavicle.

Potential Nursing Diagnoses

Impaired skin integrity related to immobility
Altered peripheral tissue perfusion related to immobility

Steps	Rationale
1. Wash hands.	Reduces transmission of micro-organisms.
2. Place client on his abdomen in center of bed.	Prepares client for proper positioning.
3. Turn client's head to side and place small pillow underneath.	Maintains proper alignment and prevents lateral flexion of neck.
4. Place a pillow under client's flexed arm. Pillow should extend from his hand to elbow. (Fig. 17)	Prevents internal rotation of shoulder.

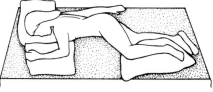

Fig. 17

95

Steps	Rationale
5. Place another pillow under his flexed leg, to extend from knee to foot.	Prevents internal rotation of hip and adduction of leg. Also reduces pressure on knees and ankles from mattress.
6. Place sandbags or foot-drop stops against client's feet.	Maintains feet in dorsiflexion. Reduces risk of foot-drop.
7. Wash your hands.	Reduces transmission of microorganisms.
8. Record in nurse's notes client's new position.	Documents that procedure was performed.

Nurse Alert

The nurse should be aware of potential trouble areas with the Sims position: lateral flexion of the neck; internal rotation, adduction, or lack of support to the shoulders and hips; foot-drop; and potential pressure sores at the ears, ilium, humerus, clavicle, knees, and ankles.

Client Teaching

The Sims position provides the nurse an opportunity to teach the family about range of joint motion and skin care. In addition, the nurse can demonstrate proper positioning measures.

Pediatric Considerations

The Sims position is used with an unconscious, immobilized, or burned child. If the child is alert, the nurse should incorporate quiet diversional activities into her care plan so the Sims position will be maintained.

Geriatric Considerations

Because of the normal aging process, an elderly client's musculoskeletal system is at risk of joint deformities, loss of muscle mass, and skin breakdown. If degenerative joint disease (osteoarthritis) is also present, the client may require his position to be changed every hour instead of every 2 hours.

Assisting a Client to Move Up in Bed (One or Two Nurses)

The nurse will frequently encounter a semi-helpless, helpless, or immobilized client whose position must be changed or who must be moved up in bed. Proper use of body mechanics can enable her (and a helper) to move, lift, or transfer such a client safely and at the same time avoid musculoskeletal injury.

Potential Nursing Diagnoses

Activity intolerance related to immobility
Impaired skin integrity related to immobility

Steps	Rationale
1. Wash hands.	Reduces transmission of micro-organisms.
2. Face head of bed. (If two nurses are assisting client, each stands at one side of bed.)	Facing direction of movement prevents twisting of your body when moving client.
3. Place your feet apart with foot nearer bed behind other foot.	Increases your balance. One foot behind other allows you to transfer your body weight as client is moved up in bed.
4. If possible, ask client to flex his knees, bringing his feet as close to buttocks as possible.	Enables client to use his leg muscles during process of actually moving up in bed.

Steps	Rationale
5. Instruct client to flex his neck, tilting chin toward chest.	Prevents hyperextension of neck when moving to head of bed.
6. Ask him to assist in moving by using trapeze bar if available or pushing on bed surface.	He uses his upper extremity muscles to elevate trunk and reduce friction when moving up in bed.
7. If client has limited upper extremity strength or mobility, place his arms across his chest.	Prevents friction from arms dragging across bed surface during move.
8. Flex your knees and hips, bringing your forearms closer to level of bed.	Increases your balance and strength by bringing your center of gravity closer to client, the "object" to be moved.
9. Place arm that is closer to head of bed under client's shoulder and other arm under client's thighs.	Prevents trauma to client's musculoskeletal system, because his shoulder and hip joints are supported. Also evenly distributes client's weight.
10. Instruct client to move up in bed on count of three.	Prepares client for actual move, thus reinforcing his assistance.
11. On count of three, rock and shift your weight from back leg to front leg. At same time, have client push with his heels and elevate his trunk. (Fig. 18)	Enables you to improve your balance and overcome inertia. Shifting your weight counteracts client's weight. When client pushes with his heels and lifts his trunk, friction is reduced.

 Fig. 18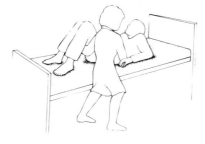

Steps	Rationale
12. Reassess client's body alignment. If poor, reposition client into proper position.	Proper body alignment increases client's comfort, promotes rest, and reduces hazards of immobility.
13. Record in nurse's notes client's new position.	Documents that procedure was performed.

Nurse Alert

The nurse must avoid dragging a client up in bed. This causes a shearing force. The shearing force causes damage to the underlying tissue capillaries and reduces blood flow to the region. Shearing also causes abrasions to the skin, resulting in peripheral thromboses, which further decreases blood flow to the area.

Client Teaching

This skill provides an excellent opportunity for the nurse to teach a client and his family how to maintain proper body alignment while moving him up in bed.

Pediatric Considerations

The nurse is usually able to pick a child up and reposition him. However, when the child is in traction, additional assistance may be needed to maintain alignment.

Geriatric Considerations

Elderly clients with degenerative joint disease (osteoarthritis) are at greater risk than younger clients of shoulder joint dislocation while being moved. In addition, their decreased muscle mass and reduced skin elasticity and skin moisture increase their risk of skin breakdown from shearing force.

Assisting a Client
to the Sitting Position

A partially immobilized or weak client will require nursing assistance to sit up in bed. The nurse can help such a client attain the sitting position while maintaining proper body alignment for herself as well as the client. Correct positioning techniques will reduce the risk of musculoskeletal injury to all persons involved.

Potential Nursing Diagnoses

Activity intolerance related to immobility
Impaired skin integrity related to immobility

Steps	Rationale
1. Wash hands.	Reduces transmission of micro-organisms.
2. Place client in supine position.	Enables you to continually assess client's body alignment and administer additional care, such as suctioning or hygiene needs.
3. Remove all pillows.	Decreases interference while sitting client up in bed.
4. Face head of bed.	Reduces twisting of your body when moving client.
5. Place your feet apart with foot nearer bed behind other foot.	Improves your balance and allows you to transfer your body weight as client is moved to sitting position.
6. Place hand that is farther from client under client's shoulders, supporting his head and cervical vertebrae.	Maintains alignment of client's head and cervical vertebrae and allows for even lifting of his upper trunk.

Steps	Rationale
7. Place your other hand on bed surface.	Provides support and balance.
8. Raise client to a sitting position by shifting your weight from front leg to back leg. (Fig. 19)	Improves your balance, overcomes inertia, and transfers your weight in direction of move.

Fig. 19

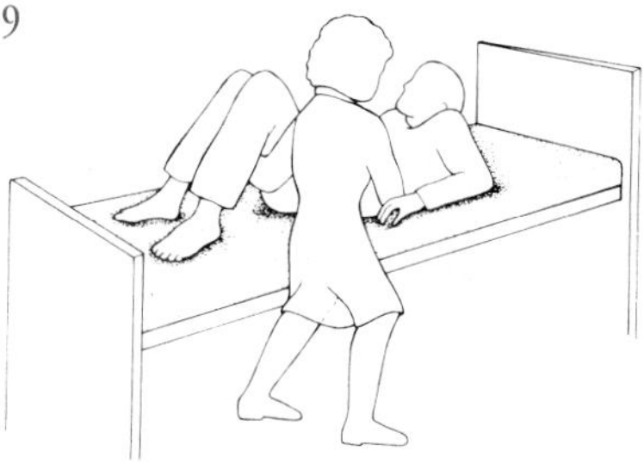

9. Push against bed and the arm that was on bed surface.	Divides activity of raising client to a sitting position between your arms and legs and protects your back from strain. By bracing one hand against mattress and pushing against it as you lift client, you transfer part of weight that would be lifted by your back muscles through your arms and onto mattress.
10. Wash hands.	Reduces transmission of microorganisms.
11. Record in nurse's notes client's new position.	Documents that procedure was performed.

Nurse Alert

The nurse must avoid dragging a client up in bed. Dragging against the bed linen causes shearing force. In addition, she should carefully observe the client for signs of the possible development of postural hypotension (dizziness, fainting, etc.).

Client Teaching

This skill provides an opportunity for the client and family to learn appropriate body alignment for the sitting position.

Pediatric Considerations

Children are usually easy to move, and the nurse may be able to simply raise a child to the sitting position.

Geriatric Considerations

Elderly clients with degenerative joint disease (osteoarthritis) are at greater risk than younger clients of shoulder joint dislocation while being moved. In addition, their decreased muscle mass and reduced skin elasticity and skin moisture increase the risk of skin breakdown from shearing force.

Assisting a Client to the Sitting Position on Side of Bed

The partially immobilized or weak client will require nursing assistance to attain a sitting position in bed. The nurse can help such a client sit up while at the same time maintaining proper body alignment for herself and the client and reducing the risk of musculoskeletal injuries to all persons involved. Frequently this is the first activity ordered for a client who has been on bedrest.

Potential Nursing Diagnoses

Activity intolerance related to immobility
Impaired skin integrity related to immobility

Steps	Rationale
1. Wash hands.	Reduces transmission of micro-organisms.
2. Place client in side-lying position, facing you on side of bed where he will be sitting. Put up side rail on opposite side.	Prepares client for move and protects him from falling.
3. Raise head of bed to highest level (or highest level that client can tolerate).	Decreases amount of work needed by you and client to raise him to sitting position.
4. Stand opposite client's hips.	Places your center of gravity nearer client.

103

Steps	Rationale
5. Turn on a diagonal so you are facing client and far corner of bed.	Reduces twisting of your body, since you are facing direction of movement.
6. Place your feet apart with foot closer to head of bed in front of other foot.	Increases your balance and allows you to transfer your weight as client is brought to sitting position at side of bed.
7. Place arm that is nearer head of bed under client's shoulders, supporting his head and neck.	Maintains alignment of client's head and neck as you bring him to sitting position.
8. Place your other arm over client's thighs. (Fig. 20)	Supports client's hip and prevents him from falling backward during procedure.
9. Move client's lower legs and feet over side of bed.	Decreases friction and resistance during the procedure.
10. Pivot toward your rear leg, allowing client's upper legs to swing downward. (Fig. 21)	Allows gravity to work with you to lower client's legs.

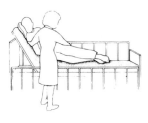

Fig. 20

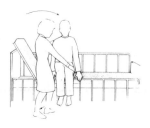

Fig. 21

11. At same time, shift your weight to rear leg and elevate client.	Allows you to transfer your weight in direction of motion.
12. Remain in front of client until he regains balance.	Reduces client's risk of falling.
13. Lower the level of bed until client's feet are touching floor.	Supports client's feet in dorsal flexion and allows client to easily stand at side of bed.

Steps	Rationale
14. Wash hands.	Reduces transmission of micro-organisms.
15. Record in nurse's notes client's new position.	Documents that procedure was performed.

Nurse Alert

Clients who have been in bed for a long period of time are at risk of postural hypotension. The nurse should assess their vital signs before placing them in a sitting position. During the procedure the nurse should assess for signs of dizziness, weakness, light-headedness, or pallor. If these symptoms develop, stop the procedure. Once the client is stable and sitting on the side of the bed, the nurse should reassess the vital signs.

Client Teaching

This skill provides the client and family an opportunity to learn the basic mechanics of appropriate body alignment for the sitting position.

Pediatric Considerations

Children usually are easy to move, and the nurse may be able to independently lift a child up in bed.

Geriatric Considerations

Elderly clients with degenerative joint disease (osteoarthritis) are at greater risk than younger clients of shoulder joint dislocation while being assisted up in bed. In addition, because of underlying cardiovascular disease, they may be at increased risk of postural hypotension.

Transferring a Client from Bed to Chair

Transferring a client from bed to chair enables the nurse to change his surroundings as well as his position. If the client is able to tolerate transfer to a wheelchair, the nurse can move him out of his room into other surroundings and increase his opportunities for socialization. For clients who have been on bedrest this is one of the first activities to be resumed.

Potential Nursing Diagnoses

Activity intolerance related to immobility
Impaired skin integrity related to immobility

Steps	Rationale
1. Wash hands.	Reduces transmission of microorganisms.
2. Assist client to a sitting position on side of bed. Have chair in position with back of chair parallel to head of bed.	Prepares client for move.
3. Place your feet apart.	Ensures better balance.
4. Flex your hips and knees, aligning your knees with client's. (Fig. 22)	Flexion of hips and knees lowers your center of gravity to level of "object" being raised. Aligning your knees with client's allows for stabilization when he stands.

Steps   Rationale

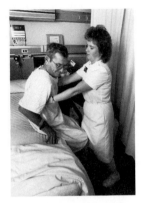

Fig. 22

5. Straighten your hips and   Uses correct body mechanics to
   legs. (Fig. 23)   raise client to a standing posi-
                                   tion.

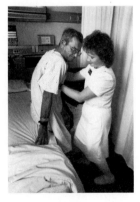

Fig. 23

Steps	Rationale
6. Pivot on foot that is farther from chair, moving client directly in front of chair. (Fig. 24)	Maintains client's support while allowing adequate space for him to move.

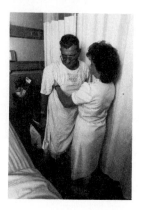

Fig. 24

Steps	Rationale
7. Instruct client to use arm-rests on chair for support.	Increases client's stability.
8. Flex your hips and knees while lowering client into chair. (Fig. 25)	Prevents injury to you resulting from poor body mechanics.

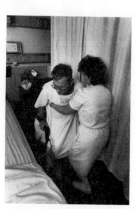

Fig. 25

Steps	Rationale
9. Assess client for proper alignment.	
10. Wash hands.	Reduces transmission of micro-organisms.
11. Record in nurse's notes client's safe transfer to chair.	Documents that procedure was performed.

Nurse Alert

Transfer of a client from bed to chair by one nurse requires assistance from the client and should not be attempted if the client is unable to help or to understand the nurse's instructions.

Client Teaching

This is an appropriate time to teach a client and his family the principles of safe transfer technique and body alignment.

Pediatric Considerations

Because children often are easier to move, the nurse may be able to independently lift a child from bed to chair. However, once the child is in the chair, the nurse must reassess his body alignment to ensure proper positioning.

Geriatric Considerations

Physiological changes of aging result in some sensory disturbances that make transferring an elderly client from bed to chair more difficult. First, the client may be increasingly susceptible to postural hypotension, dizziness, and the risk of fainting. Second, changes in his visual and hearing acuity may make it more difficult for him to accurately visualize the chair or understand instructions. Last, decreased balance and changes in the musculoskeletal system increase his risk of falling.

Crutch Walking

Crutches are often needed to increase a client's mobility. The use of crutches may be temporary (such as after ligament damage to the knee) or permanent (as with paralysis of the lower extremities). It is important that crutches be measured for the appropriate length and that clients be taught how to use them correctly.

Potential Nursing Diagnoses

Impaired physical mobility related to injured lower extremity
Potential for injury related to use of crutches
Impaired skin integrity related to axillary pressure from crutch pad

Equipment

Tape measure   Rubber crutch tips
Goniometer   Wooden crutches

Steps	Rationale
1. Wash hands.	Reduces transmission of micro-organisms.
2. Measure for crutch length: 3-4 finger widths from axilla to a point 15 cm (6 inches) lateral to client's heel. (Fig. 26)	Ensures that crutches are individualized to client's height.

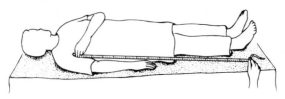

Fig. 26

Steps	Rationale
3. Position crutch handgrips with elbows flexed at 20-25 degree angle. Angle of elbow flexion should be verified by goniometer. (Fig. 27)	Prevents client's body weight from being supported by axillae and consequent nerve damage.
4. Verify that distance between crutch pad and axilla is 3-4 finger widths. (Fig. 28)	Prevents axillary skin breakdown secondary to pressure from crutch pad.

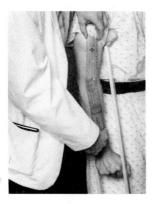

Fig. 27

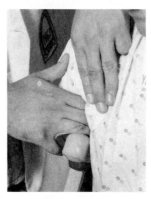

Fig. 28

5. Instruct client to assume tripod stance. Tripod stance is formed when crutches are placed 15 cm (6 inches) in front and 15 cm to side of each foot. (Fig. 29)

Improves balance by providing wider base of support. No weight should be borne by axillae.

Fig. 29

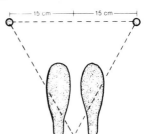

Steps	Rationale
6. Teach client one of four crutch walking gaits (Darkened areas on Figs. 30-32 represent weight-bearing):	Allows client to ambulate safely. Specific type of gait chosen depends on client's impairment and physician's order.

- ■ Four-point alternating or four-point gait gives stability to client but requires weight bearing on both legs. Each leg is moved alternately with each crutch so three points of support are on floor at all times. (Fig. 30)
- ■ Three-point alternating or three-point gait requires client to bear all weight on one foot. Weight is borne on uninvolved leg, then on both crutches, and the sequence is repeated. Affected leg does not touch ground during early phase of three-point gait. Gradually client progresses to touchdown and full weight bearing on affected leg. (Fig. 31)
- ■ Two-point gait requires at least partial weight bearing on each foot. Client moves each crutch at same time as opposing leg, so crutch movements are similar to arm motion during normal walking. (Fig. 32)
- ■ Swing-through or swing-to gait is frequently used by paraplegics who wear weight-supporting braces

Steps	Rationale

on their legs. With
weight on supported
legs, client places
crutches one stride in
front and then swings to
or through them while
they support his weight.

7. Teach client to ascend and descend on stairs: | Reduces risk of further damage to musculoskeletal system and risk of falling.

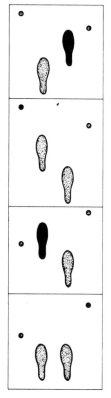

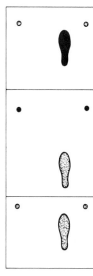

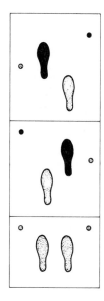

Fig. 30   Fig. 31   Fig. 32

Steps	Rationale

Ascend

- Assume a tripod position.
- Transfer body weight to crutches. (Fig. 33)
- Advance unaffected leg between crutches and stair.
- Shift weight from crutches to unaffected leg. (Fig. 34)
- Align both crutches on stair. (Fig. 35)

Descend

- Transfer body weight to unaffected leg. (Fig. 36)
- Place crutches on stair and begin to transfer body weight to crutches, moving affected leg forward. (Fig. 37)
- Align unaffected leg on stair with crutches. (Fig. 38)

8. Teach client how to sit in chair and how to get up from chair:

   Provides safe method of sitting in and getting up from chair. Reduces further damage to client's musculoskeletal system and the risk of falling.

Sitting

- Client positioned at center front of chair with posterior aspects of legs touching chair. (Fig. 39)
- Client holds both crutches in hand opposite affected leg. If both legs are affected, crutches are held in hand on client's stronger side. (Fig. 40)
- Client grasps arm of chair with remaining hand and lowers body into chair. (Fig. 41)

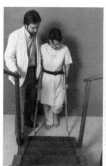
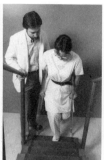
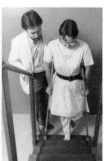

Fig. 33   Fig. 34   Fig. 35

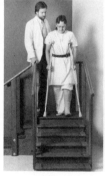
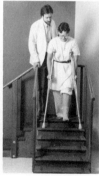
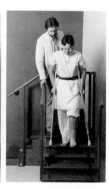

Fig. 36   Fig. 37   Fig. 38

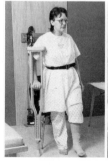
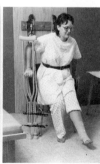
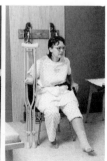

Fig. 39   Fig. 40   Fig. 41

Steps	Rationale

Getting up
- Perform three steps above in reverse order.

9. Wash hands. — Reduces transmission of micro-organisms.

10. Record in nurse's notes gait and procedures taught and client's ability to perform gaits. — Documents teaching and client's learning.

Nurse Alert

The client with cognitive impairment or who has received analgesics or tranquilizers may be unable to understand instruction or unable to safely ambulate with crutches.

Client Teaching

The nurse should instruct the client that, because of the potential for axillary skin breakdown and nerve damage, he must not lean on his crutches to support his body weight. Rubber crutch tips should be replaced as they wear out, and they should remain dry. Worn or wet crutch tips decrease surface tension and increase the risk of falling. The client should be given a list of medical suppliers in his community so he can obtain repairs as well as new rubber tips, handgrips, and crutch pads. In addition, it is advisable that he have spare crutches and tips on hand.

Geriatric Considerations

The normal visual acuity and depth perception changes with aging may prevent the client from safely ascending or descending stairs with crutches.

Applying Elastic
Stockings

Elastic stockings reduce the risk of thrombus formation. Available in toe-to-knee and toe-to-midthigh sizes, they promote venous return by maintaining pressure on the muscles of the lower extremities.

Potential Nursing Diagnoses

Altered peripheral tissue perfusion related to immobility

Equipment

Talcum powder
Basin and water
Wash cloth and towel
Tape measure
Elastic support stockings in correct size

Steps	Rationale
1. Remove elastic stockings at least twice a day.	Enables you to clean and assess skin and vessels of the legs.
2. Wash hands.	Reduces transmission of micro-organisms.
3. After legs have been cleaned, apply a small amount of talcum powder to each leg and foot.	Reduces friction and allows for easier application of stocking.

Steps	Rationale
4. Turn elastic stocking inside out down to foot by placing one hand into sock, holding toe of sock with other hand, and pulling. (Fig. 42)	Allows easier application of stocking.
5. Place client's toe into foot of elastic stocking, making sure that sock is smooth. (Fig. 43)	Wrinkles in sock can impede circulation to lower region of extremity.
6. Slide remaining portion of stocking over client's foot and heel, being sure that his toes are covered. Stocking will now be right side out. (Fig. 44)	If toes remain uncovered, they will become constricted by the elastic and their circulation can be reduced.
7. Slide stocking up over client's calf until it completely covers the leg. Be sure that it is smooth and contains no wrinkles. (Fig. 45)	Ridges impede venous return and can counteract overall purpose of elastic stocking.
8. Instruct client not to roll the stockings partially down.	Rolling sock partially down will have a constricting effect and impede venous return.
9. Wash hands.	Reduces transmission of microorganisms.
10. Record in nurses's notes removal and reapplication of elastic stockings, client's skin integrity, and adequacy of circulation to distal extremities.	Documents that procedure was performed.

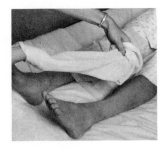

Fig. 42

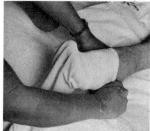

Fig. 43

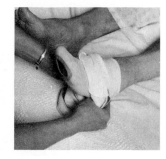

Fig. 44

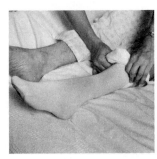

Fig. 45

Nurse Alert

Clients who wear elastic stockings must have the circulation to their distal extremities checked at least every 2 hours. The nurse evaluates the circulation by assessing capillary refill of the great toe. This is done by compressing the nail bed, observing the blanching, and noting the promptness of return to normal color (2 to 3 seconds). If capillary refill is greater than 2 or 3 seconds and the toes are cold, the elastic stockings are impeding circulation and must be removed.

Client Education

This procedure enables the nurse to teach the client good foot care as well as application of elastic stockings for his return home.

Geriatric Considerations

Elastic stockings should not be used, or should be used only with caution, in clients who have chronic peripheral vascular disease, diabetes, or chronic venous leg ulcers.

PRESSURE
ULCERS

Risk Assessment
and Prevention

A pressure ulcer, or decubitus ulcer, is an inflammation or ulcer that develops in the skin as a result of a prolonged period of ischemia in the tissues. This type of ulcer poses serious threats to a client's health. The break in the skin eliminates the body's first line of defense against infection. Ulcers that invade the subcutaneous tissues result in the loss of protein-rich and electrolyte-rich body fluids from the wound.

Nursing care requires continuous assessment of the skin and potential pressure sites (Fig. 46), meticulous hygiene, turning, and other aggressive measures to prevent pressure ulcer formation.

Potential Nursing Diagnoses

Impaired physical mobility related to musculoskeletal injury
Impaired skin integrity related to immobility
Altered peripheral tissue perfusion related to immobility

Steps	Rationale
1. Identify client's risk for decubitus ulcer formation:	Determines need to administer preventive care in addition to use of topical agents for existing ulcers.
a. Paralysis or immobilization caused by restrictive devices	Client unable to turn or reposition self independently.
b. Sensory loss	Client feels no discomfort from pressure.
c. Circulatory disorders	Disorders reduce perfusion of skin's tissue layers.

Steps	Rationale
d. Fever	Causes increase in metabolic demands of tissues. Accompanying diaphoresis leaves skin moist.
e. Anemia	Decreased hemoglobin reduces oxygen-carrying capacity of blood and amount of oxygen available to tissues.
f. Malnutrition	Inadequate nutrition can lead to weight loss, muscle atrophy, and reduced tissue mass. Less tissue is available to pad between skin and underlying bone. Poor protein, vitamin, and caloric intake limit person's wound-healing capabilities.
g. Incontinence	Skin becomes exposed to moist environment containing bacteria. Moisture causes skin maceration.
h. Heavy sedation and anesthesia	Client is not mentally alert; does not turn or change position independently. Sedation can also alter sensory perception.
i. Elderly	Skin is less elastic and drier; tissue mass is reduced.
j. Dehydration	Results in decreased elasticity and turgor.
k. Edema	Edematous tissues are less tolerant of pressure, friction, and shear force.
l. Existing pressure ulcers	Limits surfaces available for position changes, placing available tissues at increased risk.

2. Assess condition of client's skin over regions of pressure. (Fig. 46)

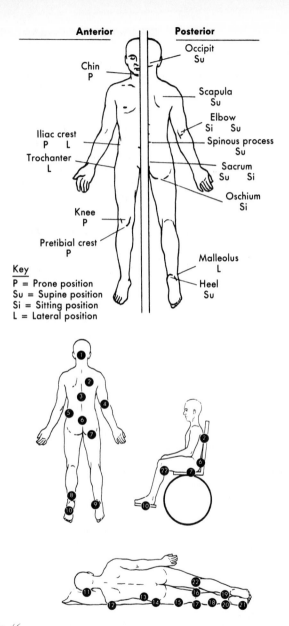

Anterior **Posterior**

Occipit
Su

Chin
P

Scapula
Su

Elbow
Si   Su

Iliac crest
P   L

Spinous process
Su

Trochanter
L

Sacrum
Su   Si

Oschium
Si

Knee
P

Pretibial crest
P

Malleolus
L

Heel
Su

Key
P = Prone position
Su = Supine position
Si = Sitting position
L = Lateral position

Fig. 46
From Trelease CC: Developing standards for wound care, Ostomy/Wound Management 20:46, 1988.

Steps	Rationale
a. Redness, warmth	May indicate tissue was under pressure, hyperemia is a normal physiological response to hypoxemia in the tissues.
b. Pallor and mottling	Persistent hypoxia in tissues that were under pressure; an abnormal physiological response.
c. Absence of superficial skin layers	Represents early pressure ulcer formation.
3. Assess client for additional areas of potential pressure, specifically:	High-risk clients have multiple sites in addition to bony prominences for pressure necrosis:
a. Nares	NG tube
b. Tongue, lips	Oral airway, ET tube
c. IV sites (especially long-term access sites)	Stress on catheter at exit site
d. Drainage tubes	Stress against tissue at exit site
e. Foley catheter	Pressure against labia, especially with edema

Key for Fig. 46

Pressure ulcer sites

1. Occipital bone
2. Scapula
3. Spinous process
4. Elbow
5. Iliac crest
6. Sacrum
7. Ischium
8. Achilles tendon
9. Heel
10. Sole
11. Ear
12. Shoulder
13. Anterior iliac spine
14. Trochanter
15. Thigh
16. Medial knee
17. Lateral knee
18. Lower leg
19. Medial malleolus
20. Lateral malleolus
21. Lateral edge of foot
22. Posterior knee

Steps	Rationale
4. Observe client for preferred positions when in bed or chair.	Weight of body will be placed on certain bony prominences. The presence of contractures may result in pressure being exerted in unexpected places. This phenomenon can be assessed best through observation.
5. Observe ability of client to initiate and assist with position changes.	Potential for friction and shear pressure increases when client is completely dependent for position changes.
6. Obtain "Risk Score" (Table 1)	Risk score will depend on the instrument used.
7. Assess client's and support persons' understanding of risks for pressure ulcers.	Provides opportunity for beginning prevention education.
8. Wash hands.	Prevents transmission of infection.
9. Close room door or bedside curtain.	Maintains client privacy.
10. Assist client to change of position: 　a. Supine 　b. Prone 　c. Side-lying 　d. 30-degree oblique	See Unit III for specifics. Avoid positions that place client directly on an area of existing ulceration. Achieved with one pillow under the shoulder and one pillow under the leg on the same side. Protects sacrum and trochanters.
11. Observe area that had been under pressure for redness.	Initial flushing is expected.

Table 1   Norton Scale

Physical Condition		Mental Condition		Activity		Mobility		Incontinent (Bowel and/or Bladder)		Total Score
Good	4	Alert	4	Ambulant	4	Full	4	Not	4	
Fair	3	Apathetic	3	Walks/help	3	Slightly limited	3	Occasional (<2 per 24 hrs)	3	
Poor	2	Confused	2	Chairbound	2	Very limited	2	Usually (>2 per 24 hrs)	2	
Very bad	1	Stupor	1	Bed	1	Immobile	1	Always	1	

From Trelease CC: Developing standards for wound care, Ostomy/Wound Management 20:46, 1988.
Maximum score = 20 (good physical condition)
Minimum score = 5
High risk for pressure ulcers = 12 or below

Steps	Rationale
12. Monitor length of time any area of redness persists. ■ Determine appropriate turning interval. ■ a turning interval of less than 1½-2 hours may not be realistic; therefore use of a pressure relief device would be recommended.	It is safe to assume redness will persist for 50% of the time hypoxia actually occurred. EXAMPLE: Turning interval 2 hours ■ Redness lasts 15 minutes. ■ Hypoxia was therefore approximately 30 minutes. ■ Recommended turning interval should be: Turning interval − hypoxia time = suggested interval ■ In this example, interval would be: 2 hours − 30 minutes = 1½ hours
13. Wash hands.	Prevents spread of microorganisms.
14. Record appearance of tissues under pressure.	Baseline observations coupled with subsequent inspections reveal success of prevention program.
15. Describe positions used, turning intervals, and other prevention measures used.	Documents care provided.

Nurse Alert

The nurse should pay special attention to body regions that receive the greatest amount of pressure in specific positions: **sitting:** ischial tuberosities and sacrum; **supine:** back of skull, elbow, sacrum, ischial tuberosities, and heels; **prone:** elbows, knees, and toes; **side-lying:** knees and greater trochanters.

Teaching Considerations

When teaching alert clients to change position for pressure relief, suggest using television programming/commercial intervals or use a watch with hourly alarm intervals.

Pediatric Considerations

The pediatric client is at risk for skin breakdown when nutritional and electrolyte impairments, fever, circulatory disorders, and incontinence are present. Also, the pediatric client with orthopedic immobilization is at risk for pressure ulcers at the cast or traction site.

Geriatric Considerations

Many older adult clients are being cared for in their homes by family members or their older adult spouse. In addition to the risks listed in Step 1, the family members need to understand that consistency must be practiced for pressure ulcer assessment and prevention.

Treatment of
Pressure Ulcers

Various topical agents have been used in the treatment of pressure ulcers. Some of these agents (e.g., astringents, alkaline soap products) have proven harmful. Beneficial agents include enzymes, antiseptics, oxidizing agents, and dry dextranomer beads.

The agent of choice depends on the depth of the ulcer. Deeper ulcers may derive greater benefit from enzyme application.

Local treatment of pressure ulcers also includes the use of a variety of dressings. The occlusive dressings are a group of dressings that are widely marketed and are being used with increasing frequency to treat pressure ulcers. The occlusive dressings (including transparent dressings, hydrocolloid dressings, and the hydrogels) may be used in combination with topical agents or by themselves.

Potential Nursing Diagnoses

Impaired skin integrity related to immobility
Impaired skin integrity related to wound secretions

Equipment

Wash basin, soap, water; cleansing agent (Table 2), or prescribed topical agents (Table 3), ordered dressings, hypoallergenic tape or adhesive dressing sheet (Hypofix), disposable or sterile gloves

Steps	Rationale
1. Wash hands and apply disposable gloves.	Reduces transmission of blood-borne pathogens. Gloves should be worn when handling items soiled by body fluids (CDC, 1987).
2. Close room door or bedside curtains.	Maintains client's privacy.

Table 2   Topical solutions

Name	Type	Comments
Acetic acid	Antimicrobial	Effective against *Pseudomonas aeruginosa*
		Discontinue use when infected organisms are gone
Biolex	Detergent	Nonionic surfactant for wound cleansing
Cara-Klenz	Detergent	Wound cleanser
Hydrogen peroxide	Oxidizing agent	Facilitates removal of necrotic debris, crusting
		Will oxidize healthy tissue—DO NOT USE in clean, healing ulcers
		Use should be discouraged in deep ulcers because gas emboli may result
Povidone-iodine	Antimicrobial	Potentially irritating to intact skin
		If used undiluted, may cause toxicity to granulating tissues
Sodium hypochlorite (Dakins)	Antimicrobial	Effective for odor control
		Protect intact skin with zinc oxide
		Discontinue use when necrotic tissue is gone

Steps	Rationale
3. Position client comfortably with area of decubitus ulcer and surrounding skin easily accessible.	Area should be accessible for cleansing of ulcer and surrounding skin.

Steps	Rationale
4. Assemble needed supplies at bedside. Open sterile packages and topical solution containers.	Sterile supplies should be ready for easy application so that nurse can use sterile gloves without contaminating them.
5. Remove bed linen and client's gown to expose ulcer and surrounding skin. Keep remaining body parts draped.	Prevents unnecessary exposure of body parts.
6. Assess pressure ulcer and surrounding skin.	
a. Note color, appearance of skin around ulcer.	Retained moisture causes maceration. Skin condition may indicate progressive tissue damage.
b. Measure diameter of pressure ulcer.	Provides an objective measure of wound size. May determine type of dressing chosen.

Table 3   Prescribed topical agents

Agent	Action
Enzymes: collagenase, fibrinolysin desoxyribonuclease, or sutilains	Proteolytic enzymes debride dead tissue to clean ulcer surface.
Antiseptics: povidone iodine, ointment or solution; merbromin, 5% or 10% solution; sodium hypochlorite, 1:12 or 1:20 solution	Antiseptic reduces bacterial growth in presence of necrotic tissue, pus, serum, or blood. Reduces infection in weeping ulcers.
Oxydizing agents: benzoyl peroxide, 20%; hydrogen peroxide, half strength	Cleans wounds, especially in presence of anaerobic bacteria. Increases oxygen supply to devitalized tissues.
Dextranomer beads: Debrisan	Cleans wounds with heavy exudate. Absorbs fluid, protein, fibrin, fibrinogen, and all products of tissue breakdown and bacterial infection.

Steps	Rationale
c. Measure depth of pressure ulcer using a sterile cotton-tipped applicator or other device that will allow a measurement of wound depth.	Depth measure is important for staging ulcer. Also assists in making volume measurement.
d. Measure depth of undermining skin by lateral tissue necrosis. Use a cotton-tipped applicator and gently probe under skin edges.	Undermining may indicate progressive tissue necrosis.
7. Wash skin surrounding ulcer gently with warm water and soap.	Cleansing of skin surface reduces number of resident bacteria.
8. Rinse area thoroughly with water.	Soap can be irritating to skin.
9. Gently dry skin thoroughly by patting lightly with towel.	Retained moisture causes maceration of skin layers.
10. Apply sterile gloves.	Aseptic technique must be maintained during cleansing, measuring, and application of dressings.
11. Cleanse ulcer thoroughly with normal saline or cleansing agent. a. Use irrigating syringe for deep ulcers. b. Cleansing may be accomplished in the shower with a hand-held shower head. c. Whirlpool treatments may be used to assist with wound cleansing and debridement.	Removes debris from wound from digested material. Previously applied enzymes may require soaking for removal.

Steps	Rationale

12. Measure wound diameters and depth.
  a. Photography, if done, should be done at a consistent distance from the wound.
  b. Tracing wound diameters may be done using transparency film.
	Provides objective record of wound size against which subsequent measurements can be compared. The Kundin Scale is an example of a tool available for wound volume calculations.

13. Apply topical agents, if prescribed:	

Enzymes

■ Keeping gloves sterile, place small amount of enzyme ointment in palm of hand. ■ Soften medication by rubbing briskly in palm of hand.	It is not necessary to apply thick layer of ointment. Thin layer absorbs and acts more effectively. Excess medication can irritate surrounding skin. Makes ointment easier to apply to ulcer.
■ Apply thin, even layer of ointment over necrotic areas of ulcer. Do not apply enzyme to surrounding skin.	Proper distribution of ointment ensures effective action. Enzyme can cause burning, paresthesia, and dermatitis to surrounding skin.
■ Moisten gauze dressing in saline and apply directly over ulcer.	Protects wound. Keeping ulcer surface moist reduces time needed for healing. Skin cells normally live in moist environment.
■ Cover moistened gauze with single dry gauze and tape securely in place.	Prevents bacteria from entering moist dressing.

Antiseptics

SUPERFICIAL ULCERS

■ Moisten sterile gauze with antiseptic solution and paint surface of ulcer.	Distributes antiseptic over entire area to effectively reduce bacterial growth.

Steps	Rationale
■ Leave ulcer open to air.	If superficial epidermal skin layer is only layer affected, keeping wound dry promotes better healing.

DEEP ULCERS

■ Apply antiseptic ointment to dominant gloved hand and spread ointment in and around ulcer.	Antiseptic ointment causes minimal tissue irritation. All surfaces of wound must be covered to effectively control bacterial growth.
■ Apply sterile gauze pad over ulcer and tape securely in place.	Protects ulcer and prevents removal of ointment during turning or repositioning.

Oxidizing Agents

■ Spread zinc oxide paste over skin surface surrounding ulcer.	Oxidizing agents can be caustic to normal tissues.
■ Apply single layer of gauze dressing moistened in oxidizing solution over the ulcer (do not apply full-strength peroxide).	Coats wound surface and retains exposure to tissue surface.
■ Apply dry gauze dressing over ulcer.	Protects ulcer and prevents loosening or pulling away of moist dressing.

Dextranomer Beads

■ Hold container of beads approximately 1 in (2.5 cm) above ulcer site and lightly sprinkle 5 mm-diameter layer over wound.	Layer of insoluble powder is needed to absorb wound exudate.
■ Apply gauze dressing over ulcer.	Holds beads in place and protects wound.

Steps	Rationale

Hydrocolloid Beads/Paste

- Fill ulcer defect to approximately one-half of the total depth with hydrocolloid beads or paste.

  Hydrocolloid beads/paste will assist in absorbing wound drainage. Highly draining wounds are best treated with hydrocolloid beads/granules.

- Cover with hydrocolloid dressing; extend dressing 1-1½ inches beyond edges of wound.

  Dressing maintains wound humidity. May be left in place up to 7 days.

Hydrogel Agents

- Cover surface of ulcer with hydrogel using sterile applicator or gloved hand.

  Provide for maintenance of wound humidity while absorbing excess drainage. May be used as a carrier for topical agents.

- Apply dry, fluffy gauze over gel to completely cover ulcer.

  Holds hydrogel against wound surface. Absorbent.

14. Reposition client comfortably off pressure ulcer.

  Avoids accidental removal of dressings.

15. Remove gloves and dispose of soiled supplies. Wash hands.

  Prevents transmission of microorganisms.

16. Report any worsening in ulcer's appearance to nurse in charge or physician.

  Worsening of condition may indicate need for additional therapy.

Nurse Alert

Early ulcers tend to have irregular borders; with time, borders become smooth and rounded. If wound is large, irrigating with plain sterile water from an irrigating syringe may be helpful.

Teaching Considerations

All individuals participating in client's wound care should be taught the correct method to administer ulcer care.

MEDICATIONS

Administering Oral Medications

The most desirable route to administer medications is by mouth. Oral medications are available in various liquid and solid forms, with each type requiring special considerations when given to a client. For example, enteric-coated tablets should never be crushed, cough syrups should never be followed by liquids, and sublingual medications should be placed under the client's tongue. Unless the client has impaired gastrointestinal functioning or is unable to swallow, an oral medication is the safest and easiest to give.

Potential Nursing Diagnoses

Knowledge deficit regarding medication administration related to inexperience

Altered health maintenance related to poor drug therapy compliance

Equipment

Medication cards, Kardex, or record form
Medication cart or tray
Disposable medication cups
Glass of water or juice
Drinking straw

Steps	Rationale
1. Assess for any contraindications for oral medication administration, history of allergies, medication history, and diet history.	Reduces risk to client with impaired swallowing or gastrointestinal functioning and medication allergies.

Steps	Rationale
2. Assess client's preference for fluids to accompany medications.	Facilitates medication administration and increases client's fluid intake.
3. Gather equipment listed on previous page.	Provides efficient and accurate medication administration.
4. Check accuracy and completeness of each card or form with physician's written medication order, looking at client's name, drug name and dosage, route of administration, and time for administration.	Physician's order is most reliable resource and the only legal record of drugs client is to receive. NOTE: Check all orders at least every 24 hours.
5. Recopy any card or portion of form that is illegible.	Cards that are soiled or illegible can be source of drug errors.
6. Wash hands.	Removal of microorganisms minimizes their transfer from your hands to medications and equipment.
7. Arrange medication tray and cups in medicine room or move medication cart to position outside client's room.	Organization of equipment saves time and reduces error.
8. Unlock medicine drawer or cart.	Medications are safeguarded when locked in cabinet or cart.
9. Prepare medications for one client at a time. Keep medication tickets or forms for each client together.	Prevents preparation errors.
10. Select correct drug from stock or unit dose drawer and compare with medication card or form.	Reading label against transcribed order reduces error.
11. Calculate correct dosage.	Calculation will be more accurate when information from drug labels is at hand.

Steps	Rationale
12. To administer tablets or capsules from bottle, pour required number into bottle cap and transfer to medication cup. *Do not touch medicines with your fingers.* Extra tablets or capsules may be returned to bottle.	Aseptic technique maintains cleanliness of drugs.
13. To prepare unit dose tablets or capsules, place packaged tablet or capsule directly into medicine cup. Do not remove wrapper.	Wrappers maintain cleanliness and identification of medications.
14. All tablets or capsules given to client at same time may be placed in one cup except for those requiring preadministration assessments (such as pulse rate and blood pressure).	Keeping medications that require preadministration assessments separate from others will make it easier to withhold those drugs if necessary.
15. If client has difficulty swallowing, grind tablets in mortar with pestle. Place tablet in bottom of mortar and mix. Continue until a smooth powder remains. Mix in a small amount of soft food.	Large tablets can be difficult to swallow. Ground tablets mixed with palatable soft food are usually easy to swallow.
16. To pour liquids, remove bottle cap and place it upside down.	Prevents contamination.
■ Hold bottle with label against palm of hand while pouring.	Spilled liquid will not soil or fade label.

Steps	Rationale
■ Hold medication cup at eye level and fill to desired mark. (Scale should be even with fluid at bottom of meniscus.) (Fig. 47)	Ensures accuracy of measurement.

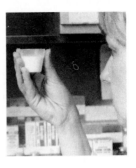

Fig. 47

Steps	Rationale
17. When preparing narcotic, check narcotic record for previous drug count, remove required volume of drug, record necessary information on form, and sign form.	Controlled substance laws require careful monitoring of dispensed narcotics.
18. Compare medication card or form with prepared drug and container.	Reading label a second time reduces error.
19. Return stock containers or unused unit-dose medications to shelf or drawer and read labels third time.	Reduces administration error.
20. Place medications and cards together on tray or cart.	Drugs are labeled at all times for identification.
21. Do not leave drugs unattended.	You are responsible for safekeeping of drugs.
22. Take medications to client at correct time.	Medications are administered within period of 30 minutes before or 30 minutes after prescribed time to ensure intended therapeutic effect.

Steps	Rationale
23. Identify client by comparing name on card or form with name on client's identification band. Ask client to state his name.	Identification bands are made at time of client's admission and are most reliable source of identification. Replace any missing ID bands.
24. Perform any necessary preadministration assessment.	Determines whether medications should be given at that time.
25. Explain purpose of medication and its action to client.	Client's understanding of purpose of medication will improve compliance with drug therapy.
26. Assist client to sitting or side-lying position.	This prevents aspiration during swallowing.
27. Administer drugs properly. Offer client choice of water or juice with drugs to be swallowed. Client may wish to hold solid medications in hand or cup before placing in mouth.	Choice of therapy promotes client comfort. Client can become familiar with medications by seeing each drug and then will be able to recognize correct drugs.
28. If client is unable to hold medications, place medication up to his lips and gently introduce drugs into his mouth.	Prevents contamination of medications.
29. If tablet or capsule falls to floor, discard it and repeat preparation.	Prevents contamination.
30. Stay with client until he has completely swallowed each medication. If uncertain whether medication was swallowed, ask client to open his mouth.	You are responsible for ensuring that client receives ordered dose. If left unattended, client may not take dose or may save drugs, causing risk to his health.
31. Wash your hands.	Reduces spread of microorganisms.

Steps	Rationale
32. Record each drug administered on medication record.	Prompt documentation prevents errors such as repeated doses.
33. Return medication cards, forms, or printouts to appropriate file for next administration time.	These are used as reference for when next dose is due. Loss of card may lead to administration error.
34. Discard used supplies, replenish stock (e.g., cups and straws), and clean work area.	Clean working space assists other staff in completing duties efficiently.
35. Return within 30 minutes to evaluate client's response to medications.	By monitoring client's response, you will assess drug's therapeutic benefit and be able to detect onset of side effects or allergic reactions.

Nurse Alert

If the client begins coughing during drug administration, stop immediately. Aspiration of medication or fluid can easily occur.

Client Teaching

Clients may require extensive instruction on how to take prescribed medications correctly. They should understand the purpose of each medication, its action and potential side effects, and the correct time and frequency of its administration. They should particularly understand what can happen if they arbitrarily increase or omit a dose or cease taking the medication entirely. They should also know whether to take medications before or after meals.

When attempting to establish medication schedules, consider the client's home environment and daily routines. Clients with visual alterations may be unable to read printed labels and thus require large-print instructions. Include family members in the teaching in case a client becomes too ill to self-administer drugs reliably.

Pediatric Considerations

Children unable to swallow or chew solid medications should be given only liquid preparations. Generally it is safe to administer solid drug forms to children 5 years or older. Pediatric preparations are usually colorful and pleasant tasting. However, a child may enjoy a "chaser" of juice, carbonated soft drink, or frozen juice bar. A bad-tasting drug can be mixed in jam, syrup, or honey. Oral medications are most easily administered to infants by spoon, plastic cup or dropper, or small plastic syringe.

Geriatric Considerations

Elderly clients often have multiple medications prescribed. It can be quite helpful to set specific time schedules convenient with their daily routines so they do not forget to take a dose. Many elderly clients have mobility and sensory limitations that prohibit safe drug preparation and administration, and family members or friends should be available for assistance.

Preparing an Injectable Medication from an Ampule

An ampule is a clear glass container with a constricted neck. It contains a single dose of a medication in liquid form. The nurse must snap off the ampule's neck to gain access to the medication. When withdrawing the medication, the nurse uses aseptic technique (by preventing the needle from touching the ampule's outer surface). Fluid can be aspirated easily into the syringe by simply drawing back on the syringe plunger.

Potential Nursing Diagnoses

This procedure may be performed by nurses caring for clients with a variety of nursing diagnoses.

Equipment

Syringe and needle of desired size
Ampule of prescribed medication
Alcohol swab or 2 × 2 gauze pad
Metal file (optional)
Extra sterile needle

Steps	Rationale
1. Wash hands.	Reduces transmission of micro-organisms.
2. Tap top of ampule lightly and quickly with a finger. (Fig. 48)	Dislodges any fluid that collects above neck. All solution moves into lower chamber.

145

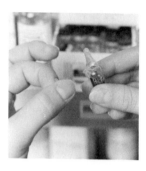

Fig. 48

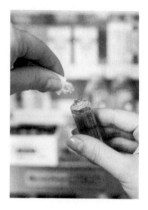

Fig. 49

Steps	Rationale
3. Partially file neck of ampule if it is not prescored.	Filing ensures a clean break.
4. Place small gauze pad or dry alcohol swab around neck of ampule.	Protects fingers from trauma as glass is broken.
5. Snap neck of ampule away from your hands. (If neck does not break, use a file to score one side of it.) (Fig. 49)	Prevents shattering glass toward your fingers or face.
6. Hold ampule either inverted or right side up. Insert needle into center of ampule opening. Do not allow needle tip or shaft to touch rim of ampule. NOTE: Ampule may be held inverted as long as needle tip or shaft does not touch its rim.	Broken rim of ampule is considered contaminated.
7. Aspirate medication into syringe by pulling back on plunger. (Fig. 50)	Withdrawal of plunger creates a negative pressure within barrel that pulls fluid into syringe.

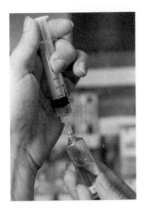

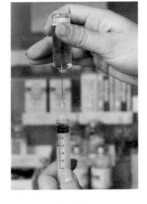

Fig. 50   Fig. 51

Steps	Rationale
8. Keep needle tip below surface of liquid. If holding ampule upright, tip it to bring all fluid within reach of needle. (Fig. 51)	Prevents aspiration of air bubbles.
9. If air bubbles are aspirated, do not expel air into ampule.	Air pressure will force fluid out of ampule, and medication will be lost.
10. To expel excess air bubbles, remove needle from ampule. Hold syringe with needle pointing up. Draw back slightly on plunger and push it upward to eject air. *Do not eject fluid.*	Withdrawing plunger too far will pull it from barrel. Holding syringe vertically allows fluid to settle in bottom of barrel. Pulling back on plunger allows fluid within needle to enter barrel.
11. After withdrawing required fluid volume, remove needle from ampule. Hold syringe and needle upright and tap syringe barrel to dislodge air bubbles. Eject air as described in Step 10.	Air within barrel displaces medication and causes dosage errors.

Steps	Rationale
12. If syringe contains excess fluid, use sink for disposal. Hold syringe vertically with needle tip up and slanted slightly toward sink. Slowly eject excess fluid into sink.	Medication is safely dispersed into sink.
Recheck fluid level by holding syringe vertically.	Rechecking fluid level ensures proper dosage.
13. Cover needle with its sheath or cap. Change needle on syringe.	Prevents contamination of needle and protects nurse from needle stick. Changing needle is required if nurse suspects medication is on needle shaft. New needle prevents tracking medication through skin and subcutaneous tissues.
14. Dispose of soiled supplies. Place broken ampule in special container for glass.	Controls transmission of infection. Proper disposal of glass prevents accidental injury to personnel.
15. Wash hands.	Reduces transmission of micro-organisms.

Nurse Alert

Use caution when snapping off the neck of an ampule. Shattering of glass can injure your hands and fingers. If you suspect that the ampule has not broken cleanly, discard and begin with a fresh ampule.

Preparing an Injectable Medication from a Vial

A vial is a single- or multiple-dose glass container with a rubber seal at the top. It can contain either a liquid or a dry drug preparation. Drugs that are unstable in solution are packaged in dry form. The vial label specifies the type of solvent used to dissolve the drug and the amount needed to prepare a desired drug concentration.

Unlike the ampule, the vial is a closed system. Air must first be injected into the vial for fluid to be easily withdrawn. Failure to inject air when withdrawing solution creates a vacuum within the vial that makes withdrawal difficult.

Potential Nursing Diagnoses

The procedure of preparing an injectable medication from a vial may be performed by nurses caring for clients with a variety of nursing diagnoses.

Equipment

Syringe and needle of desired size
Alcohol swab
Vial with prescribed medication
Extra sterile needle
Label

Steps	Rationale
1. Wash hands.	Reduces transmission of micro-organisms.

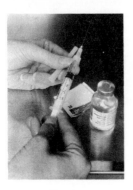

Fig. 52

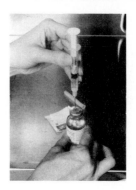

Fig. 53

Steps	Rationale
2. Remove metal cap to expose rubber seal.	Vial comes packaged with cap to prevent contamination of seal.
3. With alcohol swab, wipe off surface of rubber seal.	Removes dust or grease but does not sterilize surface.
4. Remove needle cap. Pull back on plunger to draw air into syringe equivalent to volume of medication to be aspirated. (Fig. 52)	Prevents buildup of negative pressure when aspirating medication. You must first inject air into vial.
5. Insert tip of needle, with bevel pointing up, through center of rubber seal. Apply pressure to needle point during insertion. (Fig. 53)	Center of seal is thinner and easier to penetrate. Keeping bevel up and using firm pressure prevent cutting rubber core from seal.
6. Inject air into vial, holding on to plunger.	Air must be injected first before aspirating fluid. Plunger may be forced backward by air pressure within vial.
7. Invert vial while keeping firm hold on syringe and plunger. Hold vial between thumb and middle finger of nondominant hand. Grasp end of barrel and plunger with thumb and forefinger of dominant hand.	Inverting vial allows fluid to settle in lower half of container. Position of hands prevents movement of plunger and permits easy manipulation of syringe.

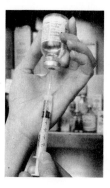

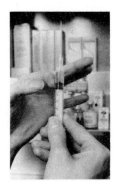

Fig. 54   Fig. 55

Steps	Rationale
8. Keep tip of needle below fluid level.	Prevents aspiration of air.
9. Allow air pressure to gradually fill syringe with medication. Pull back slightly on plunger if necessary. (Fig. 54)	Positive pressure within vial forces fluid into syringe.
10. Tap side of barrel carefully to dislodge any air bubbles. Eject any air remaining at top of syringe into vial.	Forcefully striking barrel while needle is inserted in vial may bend needle. Accumulation of air displaces medication and causes dosage errors.
11. Once correct volume is obtained, remove needle from vial by pulling back on barrel of syringe.	Pulling plunger rather than barrel causes separation from barrel and loss of medication.
12. To expel excess air bubbles, remove needle from vial by pulling back on barrel. Hold syringe with needle pointing up and tap it to dislodge bubbles. Draw back slightly on plunger and push plunger upward to eject air. *Do not eject fluid.* (Fig. 55)	Withdrawing plunger too far will pull it from barrel. Holding syringe vertically allows fluid to settle in bottom of barrel. Pulling back on plunger allows fluid within needle to enter barrel.

Steps	Rationale
13. Cover needle.	Prevents contamination of needle.
14. Change needle.	Pushing needle through rubber stopper may dull needle tip.
15. Label vial if any medication remains. Note amount of solution and concentration of drug.	Ensures accurate drug administration when successive doses are given.
16. Dispose of soiled supplies in proper containers.	Prevents transmission of infection.
17. Wash hands.	Reduces transmission of microorganisms.

Nurse Alert

Be sure that air pressure does not force the plunger out of the syringe barrel. This causes contamination of the syringe.

Mixing Two Types
of Insulin

Frequently clients with diabetes mellitus receive a combination of different types of insulin to control their blood glucose levels. Regular, rapid-acting insulin is also called unmodified insulin. This type of insulin is in a clear solution.

Other types of insulin are cloudy solutions. The cloudiness is caused by the addition of protein, which slows the absorption of the drug. These types of insulin are intermediate or long-lasting types.

When mixing two kinds of insulin, the nurse must follow two simple guidelines:

1. Regular insulin can be mixed with any other type of insulin.
2. The Lente insulins can be mixed with each other but should not be mixed with other types of insulin, except regular.

Steps	Rationale
1. Wash hands.	Reduces transmission of infection.
2. Take insulin syringe and aspirate volume of air equivalent to dosage to be withdrawn from modified insulin (cloudy vial).	Air must be introduced into vial to create pressure needed to withdraw solution.
3. Inject air into vial of modified insulin (cloudy vial). Be sure needle does not touch solution.	Prevents cross-contamination.

Steps	Rationale
4. Withdraw needle and syringe from vial and then aspirate air equivalent to dosage to be withdrawn from unmodified regular insulin (clear vial).	Air is injected into vial to withdraw desired dosage.
5. Insert needle into vial of unmodified regular insulin (clear vial), inject air, and then fill syringe with proper insulin dosage.	First portion of dosage has been prepared.
6. Withdraw needle and syringe from vial by pulling on barrel. Check dosage.	Prevents accidental pulling of plunger, which may cause loss of medication. Ensures correct dosage prepared.
7. Determine at which point on syringe scale combined units of insulin should measure.	Prevents accidental withdrawal of too much insulin from second vial.
8. Insert needle into vial of modified insulin (cloudy vial). Be careful not to push plunger and expel medication into vial. Invert vial and carefully withdraw desired amount of insulin into syringe.	Positive pressure within vial of modified insulin allows fluid to fill syringe without need to aspirate.
9. Withdraw needle and expel any excess air or fluid from syringe.	Air bubbles should not be injected into tissues. Excess fluid causes incorrect dosage.
10. Dispose of soiled supplies in proper receptacle.	Controls spread of infection.
11. Wash hands.	Reduces transmission of microorganisms.

Administering Subcutaneous and Intramuscular Injections

The administration of an injection is an invasive procedure involving deposition of medication through a sterile needle inserted into body tissues. Aseptic technique must be maintained since a client is at risk of infection once the needle penetrates the skin. The characteristics of tissues influence the rate of drug absorption and onset of drug action. Thus, before injecting a drug the nurse should know the volume of medication to administer, the characteristics of the drug, and the location of anatomical structures underlying injection sites.

For subcutaneous injections, medication is deposited into the loose connective tissue under the dermis. Since the subcutaneous tissue is not richly supplied with blood vessels, drug absorption is somewhat slower than with intramuscular injections. Subcutaneous tissues contain pain receptors so only small doses of water-soluble nonirritating medications should be given by this route.

The intramuscular route provides faster drug absorption because of a muscle's vascularity. The danger of tissue damage is less when medications enter deep muscle. Muscles also are less sensitive to irritating and viscous drugs. However, there is a risk of inadvertently injecting into a blood vessel if the nurse is not careful.

Potential Nursing Diagnoses

Potential for infection related to break in sterile technique
Pain related to injection technique

Equipment

Syringe (size varies according to volume of drug to be administered)

Needle (size varies according to type of tissue and size of client; intramuscular—20 to 23 gauge and ⅝ to 1½ inches in length; subcutaneous—25 to 27 gauge and ½ to ⅞ inch in length)

Antiseptic swab, e.g., alcohol

Medication ampule or vial

Medication card or form

Steps	Rationale
1. Wash hands.	Reduces transmission of micro-organisms.
2. Assemble equipment and check medication order for route, dose, and time.	Ensures accuracy of order.
3. Prepare medication from ampule or vial as described in Skills 5-2 and 5-3.	Ensures that medication is sterile.
4. Check client's identification band and ask client's name. Assess for allergies.	Ensures that right client receives right drug.
5. Explain procedure to client and proceed in calm manner.	Helps client anticipate nurse's actions.
6. Select appropriate injection site. Palpate site for edema, masses, or tenderness. Avoid areas of scarring, bruising, abrasion, or infection. (Fig. 56) ▪ When administering heparin subcutaneously, use abdominal injection sites. ▪ For intramuscular injection, palpate muscles to determine their firmness and size.	Injection sites should be free of lesions that might interfere with drug absorption. Sufficient muscle mass is needed to ensure accurate intramuscular injection into proper tissue. NOTE: Anticoagulants may cause local bleeding and bruising when injected into areas such as arms and legs, which are involved in muscular activity.

Fig. 56

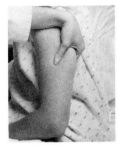

Steps	Rationale
7. In cases of repeated daily insulin injections, do not use same injection site. Rotate within a single anatomical region and then change anatomical site. Do not re-use same site within 3-week period.	Rotation of site prevents subcutaneous scarring and lipodystrophy, which can interfere with drug absorption.
8. Assist client to comfortable position depending on site chosen:	

Subcutaneous Injection

Arm—client sitting or standing
Abdomen—client sitting or supine
Leg—client sitting in bed or chair

Provides easy access to site with client in relaxed position.

Steps	Rationale

Intramuscular Injection

Thigh (vastus lateralis)—client lying supine with knee slightly flexed
Ventrogluteal—client lying on side, back, or abdomen with knee and hip on side to be injected flexed
Dorsogluteal—client prone with feet turned inward or on side with upper knee and hip flexed and placed in front of lower leg
Upper arm (deltoid)—client sitting or lying flat with lower arm flexed but relaxed across abdomen or lap

Helping client assume position that reduces strain on muscle will minimize discomfort of injection.

9. Ask client to relax his arm or leg, whichever site is chosen. Talk with him about subject of interest.

Minimizes discomfort during injection. Distraction helps reduce anxiety.

10. Relocate site using anatomical landmarks.

Accurate injection requires insertion in correct anatomical site to avoid injuring underlying nerves, bones, or blood vessels.

11. Clean the site with antiseptic swab. Apply swab at center of site and rotate outward in circular direction for about 5 cm (2 inches). (Fig. 57)

Mechanical action of swab removes secretions containing microorganisms.

12. Hold swab between third and fourth fingers of your nondominant hand.

Swab will remain readily accessible when time to withdraw needle.

13. Remove needle cap from syringe by pulling cap straight off.

Prevents needle from touching sides of cap and becoming contaminated.

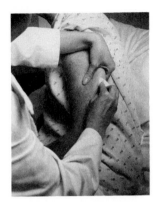

Fig. 57

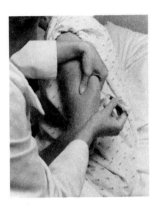

Fig. 58

Steps	Rationale
14. Hold syringe between thumb and forefinger of your dominant hand as though it were a dart. (Most nurses hold syringe palm up for subcutaneous injections and palm down for intramuscular injections because of different angles of insertion.) (Fig. 58)	Quick smooth injection requires proper manipulation of syringe parts.

15. Inject syringe:

Subcutaneous

■ For average-sized client, with your nondominant hand either spread skin tightly across injection site or pinch skin.	Needle penetrates tight skin more easily than loose skin. Pinching skin elevates subcutaneous tissue.
■ For obese client, pinch skin at site and inject needle below tissue fold.	Obese clients have fatty layer of tissue above subcutaneous tissue.
■ Inject needle quickly and firmly at a 45-degree angle. (Then release skin if pinched.)	Quick firm insertion minimizes client anxiety and discomfort.

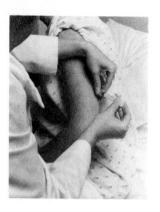

Fig. 59

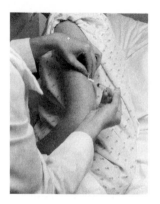

Fig. 60

Steps	Rationale

Intramuscular

- Position nondominant hand at proper anatomical landmarks and spread skin tightly. Inject needle quickly at a 90-degree angle.

  Speeds insertion and reduces discomfort.

- If muscle mass is small, grasp body of muscle and inject medication.

  Ensures that medication reaches muscle tissue.

- If giving irritating preparation, use Z-track method. Pull overlying skin and subcutaneous tissues 2.5-3.5 cm (1-1½ inches) laterally to side. Hold skin back and inject needle quickly.

  Creates zig-zag path through tissues that seals needle track to avoid tracking medication through sensitive subcutaneous tissues.

16. Once needle enters site, with your nondominant hand grasp lower end of syringe barrel. Move your dominant hand to end of plunger. Avoid movement of syringe. (Fig. 59)

    Properly performed injection requires smooth manipulation of syringe parts. Movement of syringe may displace needle and cause discomfort.

Steps	Rationale
■ If giving Z-track, keep tight hold of skin with nondominant hand. Use dominant hand to carefully move toward plunger.	Skin must remain pulled until drug injected.
17. Slowly pull back on plunger to aspirate medication. If blood appears in syringe, withdraw needle, dispose of syringe, and repeat medication preparation. If no blood appears, inject medication slowly. NOTE: Some agencies recommend not aspirating subcutaneous heparin injections.	Aspiration of blood into syringe indicates intravenous placement of needle. Subcutaneous and intramuscular medications are not for intravenous use. Slow injection reduces pain and tissue trauma. NOTE: Heparin is an anticoagulant that is typically given in small subcutaneous doses. The drug may cause bruising when aspirated. The drug is not harmful if given intravenously.
18. Withdraw needle quickly while placing antiseptic swab just above injection site. (Fig. 60)	Support of tissues around the injection site minimizes discomfort during needle withdrawal.
■ When using Z-track, keep needle inserted after injecting drug for 10 sec. Then release skin after withdrawing needle.	Allows medication to disperse evenly. Tissue planes slide across one another to create zigzag path that seals medication into muscle tissues.
19. Massage site lightly.	Massage stimulates circulation and thus improves drug distribution and absorption.
20. Assist client to a comfortable position.	Gives client sense of well-being.
21. Discard needle and syringe into appropriately labeled receptacles.	Prevents injury to client and hospital personnel. Capping needle can cause needle stick.
22. Wash hands.	Controls spread of infection.

Steps	Rationale
23. Chart medication in medication sheet or nurse's notes.	Documents administration of drug and prevents future drug errors.
24. Return to evaluate client's response to medication within 15-30 minutes.	Parenteral drugs are absorbed and act more quickly than oral medications. Your observations determine efficacy of drug action.

Nurse Alert

The needle of the syringe must remain sterile before insertion. During aspiration if blood appears in the syringe, immediately withdraw and start over. Document and report any sudden localized pain or burning at the injection site, which may indicate nerve injury.

Client Teaching

The insulin-dependent client may have to learn how to self-administer injections if family members are not available. It may be necessary to teach him aseptic principles, the basic pharmacology of insulin, the selection and rotation of injection sites, and injection techniques.

Pediatric Considerations

When it is essential to deliver a prescribed volume of solution to a child, draw up 0.2 ml of air into the syringe after preparing the drug dose. Air acts as dead space to clear the needle bore of medication. Give parents the option of helping to restrain their child during an injection. Some parents do not wish to be looked upon as the ones causing the child discomfort. It may help to keep the needle out of the child's line of vision to minimize anxiety. Never surprise a child. Be sure that he knows he is to receive an injection. The vastus lateralis is the preferred injection site for children. After the injection, provide comfort to the child.

Geriatric Considerations

The elderly client's muscle mass may be reduced. It is therefore important to choose a proper-sized needle. Remember also that the elderly client may be unable to tolerate more than 2 ml of an intramuscular injection.

Adding Medications to an Intravenous Fluid Container

The safest method for administering intravenous medications is to add the drugs to large-volume fluid containers (usually with dextrose and water solution or normal saline). Then the medication infuses slowly, the risk of side effects is minimized, and therapeutic blood levels are maintained. Drugs added to intravenous fluid containers include electrolytes, vitamins, and minerals. The primary risk involved with infusing drugs by this method is fluid overload.

Potential Nursing Diagnoses

Potential for injury related to unsafe administration of IV medications

Fluid volume excess related to IV fluids

Potential for infection related to break in sterile technique

Equipment

Prepared medication in syringe

Intravenous fluid container (bag or bottle, 500 or 1000 ml volume)

Alcohol or antiseptic swab

Label to attach to IV bag or bottle

Steps	Rationale
Adding Medication to New Container	
1. Wash hands.	Reduces transmission of micro-organisms.
2. Explain procedure to client.	Reduces client anxiety.
3. Check client's identification by reading his ID band and asking his name.	Ensures that right client gets prescribed medication.

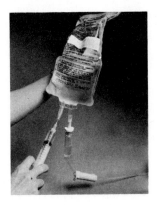

Fig. 61

Steps	Rationale
BAG	
4. Locate medication injection port on intravenous fluid bag.	The medication injection port is self-sealing to prevent introduction of microorganisms after repeated use.
5. Wipe off port with alcohol or antiseptic swab.	Reduces risk of introducing microorganisms into bag during needle insertion.
6. Carefully insert needle of syringe through center of injection port and depress plunger. (Fig. 61)	Injection of needle into sides of port may produce leak and lead to contamination of fluid.
7. Withdraw syringe and mix solution by holding the bag and turning it gently from end to end.	Allows medication to be distributed evenly throughout bag.
8. Hang bag and check infusion rate.	Prevents rapid infusion of fluid.
9. Complete medication label and stick it upside down on bag.	Label can be easily read during infusion. It alerts nurses to drug in bag.
BOTTLE	
4. Remove metal or plastic cap and rubber disk. Place cap upside down on counter top.	Cap seals bottle to maintain its sterility. Inside of cap may remain sterile for reuse.

Steps	Rationale
5. Locate medication injection site on bottle's rubber stopper. Site is usually marked by "X" or circle. Air vent and main tubing port are not injection sites.	Accidental injection through main tubing port or air vent can alter pressure within bottle and cause fluid leaks through air vent.
6. Perform Steps 5 through 9 above.	

Adding Medication to Existing Container
VENTED BOTTLE OR PLASTIC BAG

1. Check volume of solution remaining in container.	Proper volume is needed to adequately dilute medication.
2. Close off IV infusion clamp.	Prevents medication from directly entering client's circulation during injection.
3. Wipe off medication port with alcohol or antiseptic swab.	Mechanically removes microorganisms that could enter container during needle insertion.
4. Insert syringe needle through port and inject medication. (Fig. 62)	Injection port is self-sealing and prevents fluid leaks.
5. Lower container from IV pole and gently mix.	Ensures that medication is evenly distributed throughout bag.

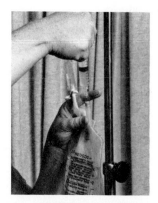

Fig. 62

Steps	Rationale
6. Rehang and regulate infusion to desired rate.	Prevents rapid infusion of fluid.
7. Label container with name and dosage of medication.	Alerts other nurses to drug in bag.

Nurse Alert

Be aware of the signs and symptoms of fluid overload in case you discover that an excess amount of fluid has infused too quickly. These include tachycardia, bounding pulse, jugular venous distention, and shortness of breath.

Client Teaching

To prevent unnecessary anxiety, the nurse should explain to the client that medications are being added to an existing IV line.

Pediatric Considerations

Infants and children are very susceptible to fluid overload, so infusions must be frequently monitored.

Geriatric Considerations

Although the conditions of renal and heart failure are not limited to the elderly population, it is especially important to consider these clients' risk for fluid overload.

Administering a Medication by Intravenous Bolus

Administration of concentrated medications directly into a vein by the bolus technique is the most dangerous method for drug administration. Drugs act rapidly since they directly enter the client's circulation. Serious side effects can occur within seconds. Therefore it is imperative that the nurse time the administrations carefully to prevent too rapid an infusion. Drugs may be given intravenously through a heparin lock or an existing intravenous infusion line. Intravenous drugs are often given by bolus in emergency situations when rapid actions are desired. The technique is also used to avoid mixing medications that are incompatible.

Potential Nursing Diagnoses

Potential for injury related to administration of IV bolus

Pain related to infiltration or needle displacement (indicates need to change IV site before drug administration)

Equipment

Heparin Lock

Prepared medication in syringe with small-gauge (25 or 26) needle

Syringe containing 1 ml of 1:1000 heparin solution (optional) or 9 ml normal saline

Alcohol or antiseptic swab

Watch with second hand or digital readout

Sterile 21- and 25-gauge needles

Medication card or form

Intravenous Infusion Line

Prepared medication in syringe with small-gauge (25 or 26) nee-
  dle
Alcohol or antiseptic swab
Intravenous line tubing with injection port
Watch with second hand or digital readout
Medication card or form

Steps	Rationale
1. Wash hands.	Reduces transmission of infection.
2. Explain procedure to client.	Reduces any anxiety client may have.
3. Check client's identification by reading identification band and asking client's name.	Ensures that right client receives right medication.

Heparin Lock

4. Clean hep lock's rubber diaphragm with antiseptic swab.	Prevents introduction of micro-organisms during needle insertion.
5. Insert 25-gauge needle of syringe containing prepared drug through center of diaphragm. (Fig. 63)	Prevents damage to diaphragm and subsequent leakage.
6. Inject medication bolus slowly over several minutes. (Each medication has recommended rate for bolus administration. Check package directions.) Use watch to time administration.	Rapid injection could prove fatal to client.

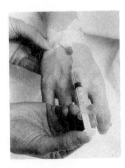

Fig. 63

Steps	Rationale
7. After administering bolus, withdraw syringe. Insert 25-gauge needle of syringe containing diluted heparin (heparin flush) or normal saline solution. Inject this.	Maintains patency of needle by inhibiting clot formation. Dilution of heparin solution prevents systemic anticoagulation of client.
8. Observe client closely for any adverse reactions.	IV medications act rapidly.
9. Dispose of syringe and needle in proper receptacle.	Prevents accidental injury from needle sticks.
10. Wash hands.	Reduces transmission of microorganisms.
11. Record in medication record drug administered.	Prompt documentation prevents drug errors.

Intravenous Infusion Line

1. Determine if IV fluids are infusing at proper rate.	Infusion must be at prescribed rate for therapeutic effect.
2. Select injection port of tubing closest to needle insertion site. (Fig. 64)	Allows for easier fluid aspiration to obtain blood return.
3. Clean off injection port with antiseptic swab.	Prevents introduction of microorganisms during needle insertion.
4. Insert small-gauge needle containing prepared drug through center of port. (Fig. 65)	Prevents damage to port's diaphragm and subsequent leakage.

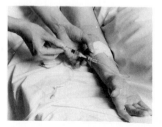

Fig. 64   Fig. 65

Steps	Rationale
5. Occlude intravenous line by pinching tubing just above injection port. Pull back gently on syringe's plunger to aspirate for blood return. (Fig. 66)	Ensures that medication is being delivered into bloodstream.
6. After noting blood return, release tubing and inject medication slowly over several minutes. (Read directions on drug package.) Use a watch to time administration. (Fig. 67)	Allows slow infusion of fluids. Rapid injection could prove fatal to client.
7. After injecting medication, withdraw syringe and recheck infusion rate.	Injection of bolus may alter rate of fluid infusion. Rapid infusion can cause circulatory overload.
8. Dispose of needle and syringe in proper receptacles.	Prevents accidental needle sticks and reduces transfer of infection.
9. Observe client closely for adverse reactions.	IV bolus medications act rapidly.
10. Wash your hands.	Reduces transfer of microorganisms.
11. Record in medication record drug administered.	Prompt documentation prevents drug errors.

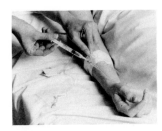

Fig. 66

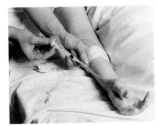

Fig. 67

Nurse Alert

Watch the IV site during drug infusion. The sudden development of swelling indicates infiltration. Then it is imperative to stop the injection. It is also imperative to know each drug's side effects and to watch the client for any reaction.

Client Teaching

The nurse may wish to inform a client on the anticipated effects of a medication. For example, an analgesic can bring rapid pain relief and it may help to encourage the client that his discomfort will soon be lessened.

Pediatric Considerations

Remember, an infant's veins are small and fragile. Rapid injection can cause infiltration.

Geriatric Considerations

An elderly client's veins are generally more fragile than a younger client's, and infiltration may occur if fluid is forced too rapidly.

Administering an Intravenous Medication by "Piggyback" or Small-Volume Container

With administration of intravenous medications through piggy-back or small-volume containers, there is less risk of causing sudden drug side effects. Medications infuse slowly over several minutes. This technique also prevents the need to infuse large volumes of fluid for clients who have fluid restrictions. The piggyback technique also avoids the need to mix drugs with others that may be incompatible. It is important that the existing intravenous line be infusing properly to ensure proper drug distribution.

Potential Nursing Diagnoses

Pain at IV insertion site related to phlebitis or infiltration
Potential for injury related to administration of IV medications
Potential for infection related to break in sterile technique

Equipment
Infusion through Adjacent Line

Medication prepared in a 50 or 100 ml infusion bag with IV infusion tubing set
Main IV infusion line
Needle (21 or 23 gauge)
Alcohol or antiseptic swab

Infusion through Volutrol

Volutrol (plastic graduated container that is part of a main IV line
  and hangs between main IV bag or bottle and infusion tubing)
Syringe with prepared medication
Alcohol or antiseptic swab
Medication label

Steps	Rationale
1. Review physician's orders for name of drug and dosage.	Ensures safe and accurate drug administration.
2. Wash hands.	Reduces transmission of micro-organisms.
3. Check client's identification band and ask client's name.	Ensures that right client receives right medication.

Piggyback Infusion through Adjacent Line

1. Prepare secondary infusion line, being sure tubing is completely filled with medication-fluid mixture.	Prevents introduction of air into main IV line.
2. Check infusion rate of main IV line.	Checking infusion rate determines patency of system. Any obstruction to flow will interfere with medication delivery.
3. Hang secondary fluid bag at or above level of main fluid bag.	Height of fluid bag regulates rate of fluid flow to client.
4. Connect needle to the end of secondary line tubing. Clean injection port to main IV line with an antiseptic swab.	Prevents introduction of micro-organisms during needle insertion.
5. Insert needle of secondary line through injection port of main IV line. Regulate flow rate of medication solution (usually 30 to 60 min).	Provides direct route for slow intermittent medication infusion. For optimal therapeutic effect, drug should infuse within 30-60 minutes.
6. Observe client for signs of adverse reactions.	IV medications act rapidly.

Steps	Rationale
7. After medication has infused, turn off flow regulator on secondary IV line. Leave needle, tubing, and secondary bag hanging for future drug administration.	Secondary line is route for microorganisms to enter main line. Repeated changes of tubing or needle increase risk of infection transmission.
8. Record in medication record drug administered.	Prompt documentation prevents drug errors.

Infusion through Volutrol

1. Check infusion rate of IV line.	Determines patency of system. Obstruction to flow interferes with medication delivery.
2. Fill Volutrol with desired amount of fluid (50-100 ml) by opening clamp between Volutrol and main IV bag. (Fig. 68)	Small volume of fluid dilutes IV medication and reduces risk of rapid dose infusion.
3. Clean off injection port on top of Volutrol.	Prevents introduction of microorganisms during needle insertion.
4. Insert syringe needle into port and inject medication. (Fig. 69) Gently rotate Volutrol between your hands.	Mixes medication within Volutrol to ensure equal distribution.

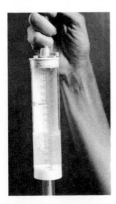
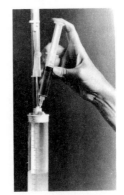

Steps	Rationale
5. Recheck IV infusion rate (medication should infuse in 30 to 60 minutes.	For optimal therapeutic effect drug should infuse within 30 to 60 minutes.
6. Wash hands.	Reduces transmission of micro-organisms.
7. Observe client for signs of adverse reactions.	IV medications act rapidly.
8. Record drug administered in medication record.	Prompt documentation prevents drug errors.
9. After medication has infused, refill Volutrol with intravenous solution and monitor flow rate as ordered.	Keeps IV line patent.

Nurse Alert

Know the potential side effects of a medication. Drugs can act rapidly.

Client Teaching

Explain the purpose and actions of a medication to the client.

Pediatric Considerations

Pediatric doses are small. Be sure that the child receives the medication in the Volutrol as well as that in the tubing. An infant or child may not receive as much infusion as an adult because of the risk of fluid overload.

Geriatric Considerations

The veins of an elderly client are fragile. Infiltration at the IV site can develop easily. Observe the site periodically during any intermittent drug infusion.

Topical Skin

Applications

A variety of pharmacological preparations can be applied to the client's skin for several purposes: maintaining hydration of skin layers, protecting skin surfaces, reducing local skin irritation, creating local anesthesia, or treating infections, abrasions, or irritations.

Although each preparation is applied in a specific manner, the nurse should be aware that these applications can create both systemic and local effects. These preparation should be applied with gloves and applicators. When an open wound is present, the use of sterile techniques is crucial.

The application of these preparations enables the nurse to thoroughly assess the client's skin and document any changes in the client's skin integrity.

Potential Nursing Diagnoses

Impaired skin integrity related to immobility
Potential impaired skin integrity related to immobility
Pain related to skin irritation
Body-image disturbance related to application of topical medications

Equipment

Ordered topical agent (e.g., cream, lotion, aerosol, spray, powder)
Medication ticket or form
Small sterile gauze dressings
Disposable or sterile gloves (optional)
Cotton-tipped applicator or tongue blade
Basin with warm water, washcloth, towel, and nondrying soap
Gauze dressings, plastic wrap, tape

Steps	Rationale
1. Review physician's order for name of drug, strength, time of administration, and site of application.	Ensures that drug will be administered safely and accurately.
2. Wash hands.	Reduces transmission of infection.
3. Arrange supplies at client's bedside.	Topical agents are not usually premeasured in medication room.
4. Close room curtain or door.	Provides for client privacy.
5. Check client's identification by reading ID bracelet and asking client's name.	Ensures that right client receives prescribed medication.
6. Position client comfortably. Remove gown or bed linen, keeping unaffected areas draped.	Provides for easy access to area being treated. Promotes client comfort.
7. Inspect condition of client's skin thoroughly. Wash any affected area, removing all debris and crustations. (Use mild nondrying soap.)	Provides baseline to determine change in skin's condition following therapy. Skin should be clean for a proper assessment. Removal of debris enhances penetration of topical drug through skin. Cleaning removes microorganisms resident in debris.
8. Pat skin dry or allow area to air dry.	Excess moisture can interfere with even application of topical agent.
9. If skin is excessively dry and flaking, apply topical agent while still damp.	Retains moisture within skin layers.
10. Don gloves if indicated.	Sterile gloves are used when applying agents to open noninfected skin lesions. Disposable gloves prevent cross-contamination of infected or contagious lesions.
11. Apply topical agent:	

Steps	Rationale

Cream, Ointment, and Oil-Based Lotion

- Place 1-2 teaspoons of medication in palm and soften by rubbing briskly between hands.

  Softening a topical agent makes it easier to apply to skin.

- Once medication is thin and smooth, smear it evenly over skin surface using long even strokes that follow direction of hair growth.

  Ensures even distribution of medication. Prevents irritation of hair follicles.

- Explain to client that skin may feel greasy after application.

  Ointments often contain oils.

Antianginal (Nitroglycerine) Ointment

- Apply desired number of inches of ointment over paper measuring guide. (Fig. 70)

  Ensures correct dosage of medication. Medication is applied to back of guide. This ensures that name and dosage of medication is readable once applied to client's skin.

- Don disposable glove if desired. Apply ointment to skin surface by holding edge or back of paper wrapper and placing ointment and wrapper directly on skin. Do not rub or massage ointment into skin. (Fig. 71)

  Drug can absorb through your fingertips, causing serious systemic effects. Medication is designed to absorb slowly over several hours and should not be massaged.

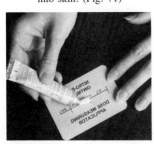

Fig. 70

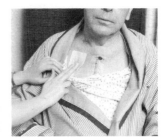

Fig. 71

Steps	Rationale
▪ Cover ointment and paper with plastic wrap and tape securely (optional).	Prevents soiling of clothing.

Aerosol Spray

▪ Shake container vigorously.	Mixes contents and propellant to ensure distribution of fine even spray.
▪ Read label for distance recommended to hold spray away from area (usually 6-12 inches)	Proper distance ensures that fine spray hits skin surface. Holding container too close results in thin watery distribution.
▪ If neck or upper chest is to be sprayed, ask client to turn face away from spray.	Prevents inhalation of spray.
▪ Spray medication evenly over affected site (in some cases spray is timed for select period of seconds).	Entire affected area of skin should be covered with thin spray.

Suspension-Based Lotion

▪ Shake container vigorously.	Mixes powder throughout liquid to form well-mixed suspension.
▪ Apply small amount of lotion to small gauze dressing or pad and apply to skin by stroking evenly in direction of hair growth.	Method leaves protective film of powder on skin after water base of suspension dries. Prevents irritation to hair follicles.
▪ Explain to client that area will feel cool and dry.	Water evaporates to leave thin layer of powder.

Powder

▪ Be sure that skin surface is thoroughly dry.	Minimizes caking and crusting of powder.

Steps	Rationale
■ Fully spread apart any skin folds such as between toes or under arms.	Fully exposes skin surface for application.
■ Dust skin site lightly with dispenser so area is covered with fine thin layer of powder.	Thin layer of powder is more absorbent and reduces friction by increasing area of moisture evaporation (Anders, 1982).
12. Cover skin area with dressing if ordered by physician.	May help prevent agent from being rubbed off skin.
13. Assist client to comfortable position, reapply gown, and cover with bed linen as desired.	Provides for client's sense of well-being.
14. Dispose of soiled supplies in proper receptacle and wash hands.	Keeps client's environment neat and reduces transmission of infection.

Nurse Alert

When applying nitroglycerine pastes, the nurse should avoid markedly hairy regions that might alter drug absorption. Antianginal creams are ordered in inches and can be measured in small sheets of paper marked in one-half inch markings.

Assess the client for allergy to topical agents. Avoid patting or rubbing skin when applying creams, ointments, or lotions. This can cause skin irritation.

Client Teaching

Assess the client's knowledge of action and purposes of medication. Determine if the client is physically able to apply medication. Caution the client against using too much of a medication since a buildup on the skin interferes with drug absorption. Be sure that the client knows the signs of local reaction to a topical agent.

Pediatric Considerations

When applying topical agents to a young child's skin, it is often necessary to cover the affected area with a dry dressing. Otherwise he may try to rub the medication off.

Geriatric Considerations

The elderly client's skin can be thin and fragile. Apply any topical agent carefully to avoid breaks in the skin. To prevent tape burns, use tape sparingly.

Administering an Eye Medication

The eye is a very sensitive organ. The cornea, or anterior portion of the eyeball, is richly supplied with sensitive pain fibers. The nurse should avoid instilling drops directly onto the corneal surface, so client discomfort will be minimal. It is also important that the nurse use caution in administering eye medications so the applicator does not accidentally touch the eye's surface. Injury can occur easily.

Eye medications are given to dilate the pupil for examination of internal eye structures, to paralyze lens muscles for measurement of lens refraction, to relieve local irritation, to treat eye disorders, and to lubricate the cornea and conjunctiva.

Potential Nursing Diagnoses

Sensory/perceptual alterations related to visual impairment

Potential for injury related to inappropriate use of eye dropper

Knowledge deficit regarding drug administration related to inexperience

Pain related to eye irritation

Equipment

Medication bottle with sterile eye dropper or ointment tube
Medication card or form
Cotton ball or tissue
Wash basin with warm water
Eye patch (optional)
Gloves

Steps	Rationale
1. Review physician's order for name of drug, dose, time of administration, and route.	Ensures safe and accurate administration of drug.

183

Steps	Rationale
2. Wash your hands and don gloves.	Reduces transfer of microorganisms.
3. Check client's identification band and ask client's name.	Ensures that right client receives right medication.
4. Explain procedure to client.	Reduces client's anxiety.
5. Ask client to lie supine with neck slightly hyperextended.	Provides easy access to eye for medication instillation. Also minimizes drainage of medication through tear duct.
6. If crusts or drainage are present along eyelid margins or inner canthus, gently wash away. Soak any crusts that are dried and difficult to remove by applying damp washcloth or cotton ball over eye for few min. Always wipe clean from inner to outer canthus.	Crusts or drainage harbor microorganisms. Soaking allows easy removal and prevents pressure from being applied directly over eye. Cleansing from inner to outer canthus avoids entrance of microorganisms into lacrimal duct.
7. Hold cotton ball or clean tissue in nondominant hand on client's cheekbone just below lower eyelid.	Cotton or tissue absorbs medication that escapes eye.
8. With tissue or cotton resting below lower lid, gently press downward with thumb or forefinger against bony orbit.	Technique exposes lower conjunctival sac. Retraction against bony orbit prevents pressure and trauma to eyeball and prevents fingers from touching eye.
9. Ask client to look at ceiling.	Action retracts sensitive cornea up and away from conjunctiva and reduces stimulation of blink reflex.

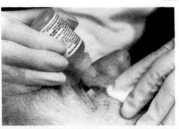

Fig. 72

Steps	Rationale
10. Instill eyedrops:	
a. With dominant hand resting on client's forehead, hold filled medication eye dropper approximately 1-2 cm (0.5-0.75 inches) above conjunctival sac. (Fig. 72)	Helps prevent accidental contact of eyedropper with eye structures, thus reducing risk of injury to eye and transfer of infection to dropper. Ophthalmic medications are sterilized.
b. Drop prescribed number of medication drops into conjunctival sac.	Conjunctival sac normally holds 1-2 drops. Applying drops to sac provides even distribution of medication across eye.
c. If client blinks or closes eye or if drops land on outer lid margins, repeat procedure.	Therapeutic effect of drug obtained only when drops enter conjunctival sac.
d. When administering drugs that cause systemic effects, protect your finger with gloves or clean tissue and apply gentle pressure to client's nasolacrimal duct for 30-60 seconds.	Prevents overflow of medication into nasal and pharyngeal passages. Prevents absorption into systemic circulation.
e. After instilling drops, ask client to close eye gently.	Helps to distribute medication. Squinting or squeezing of eyelids forces medication from conjunctival sac.
11. Instill eye ointment:	
a. Holding ointment applicator above lid margin, apply thin stream of ointment evenly along inside edge of lower eyelid on conjunctiva. (Fig. 73)	Distributes medication evenly across eye and lid margin.

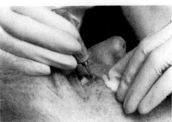

Fig. 73

Steps	Rationale
b. Ask client to look down.	Reduces blinking reflex during ointment application.
c. Apply thin stream of ointment along upper lid margin on inner conjunctiva.	Distributes medication evenly across eye and lid margin.
d. Have client close eye and rub lid lightly in circular motion with cotton ball.	Further distributes medication without traumatizing eye.
12. If excess medication is on eyelid, gently wipe it from inner to outer canthus.	Promotes comfort and prevents trauma to eye.
13. If client had eye patch, apply clean one by placing it over affected eye so entire eye is covered. Tape securely without applying pressure to eye.	Clean eye patch reduces chance of infection.
14. Wash hands and dispose of supplies.	Reduces transmission of microorganisms.

Nurse Alert

To avoid systemic side effects of certain medications, be sure to occlude the nasolacrimal duct (at the inner canthus) after administration.

Client Teaching

It may be necessary to instruct a client who is to receive an eye medication on the technique of self-administration. A client with glaucoma will usually receive medications permanently for control of this disease. Family members should also be taught proper administration techniques, especially after eye surgery when a client's vision is blurred and he has difficulty assembling supplies and handling applicators.

Warn a client against touching eye structures with the applicator. He also should know that preparations are sterile and that they should never be used if prescribed for another family member. It is common for certain medications to cause temporary blurring of vision, and the client should be warned of this.

Pediatric Considerations

A child can easily be frightened when receiving an eye medication. Talk gently with the infant or young child and be sure to restrain his head to prevent movement during instillation. A sudden twist of the head can cause the applicator to accidentally strike the eye. It is also helpful to have the hand that holds the dropper rest on the child's forehead so the hand moves synchronously with the head.

Geriatric Considerations

An elderly client with severe visual alterations will be unable to read labels of prepared medications. Certain clients may learn to recognize containers by their size and shape. However, a family member should be familiar with dose schedules and instillation techniques. A client with motor tremors may not be able to administer drugs safely.

Administering an
Inhalant

Inhaled or metered dose medications are becoming more popular. Medications administered through inhalers are dispersed through aerosol spray, mist, or fine powder to penetrate airways. Although these medications are designed to produce local effects (e.g., bronchodilator or to liquefy secretions), the medication is absorbed rapidly through the pulmonary circulation and can create systemic effects. For example, isoproterenol (Isuprel) is a bronchodilator, but it also can cause cardiac arrhythmias.

Clients with chronic lung disease often depend on metered dose inhalers to control their airway symptoms. Improper use of these medications is a common problem when clients have recurrent symptoms.

Potential Nursing Diagnoses

Ineffective airway clearance related to excess secretions
Ineffective breathing patterns related to airway constriction
Knowledge deficit regarding use of inhalant related to inexperience
Noncompliance related to improper administration of inhalant

Equipment

Metered dose inhaler with medication canister
Aerochamber (optional)
Tissues (optional)
Water for rinsing mouth, especially with steroid inhalers

Steps	Rationale
1. Allow client an opportunity to manipulate inhaler and canister. Explain and demonstrate how canister fits into inhaler.	Client must be familiar with how to use equipment.
2. Explain what a metered dose is and warn client about overuse of inhaler, including drug side effects.	Client must not arbitrarily decide to administer excessive inhalations due to risk of serious side effects. If drug is given in recommended doses, side effects are uncommon.
3. Explain steps used to administer an inhaled dose of medication (demonstrate steps when possible): ■ Remove mouthpiece cover from inhaler. ■ Shake inhaler. ■ With lips open, place inhaler in mouth. Opening should be directed toward back of throat.	Use of simple step-by-step explanations allows client to ask questions at any point during procedure. You cannot demonstrate actual depression of canister without self-administering a dose.

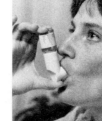

Fig. 74

■ Exhale fully. Then grasp mouthpiece with teeth and lips. (Fig. 74)	Medication should not escape through mouth.
■ While inhaling slowly and deeply through the mouth, depress medication canister fully.	Medication is distributed to airways during inhalation. Inhalation through mouth draws medication more effectively into airways.
■ Hold breath for approximately 10 seconds.	Allows tiny drops of aerosol spray to reach deeper branches of airways.
■ Then exhale through pursed lips.	Keeps small airways open during exhalation.

Steps	Rationale

4. Explain steps to administer inhaled dose of medication using aerochamber, (demonstrate when possible):

   a. Remove mouthpiece cover from metered dose inhaler and mouthpiece of aerochamber.

     Inhaler fits into end of aerochamber.

   b. Insert mouthpiece of metered dose inhaler into end of aerochamber. (Fig. 75)

     Aerochamber is a spacer that extends the distance between the inhaler and the client's mouth.

   c. Shake inhaler well.

     Ensures fine particles are aerosolized.

   d. Place aerochamber mouthpiece in mouth and close lips. Do not go beyond raised lip on mouthpiece. Avoid covering small exhalation slots with the lips.

     Medication should not escape through mouth.

   e. Breath normally through aerochamber mouthpiece.

     Allows client to relax before delivering medication.

   f. Depress medication canister, spraying one puff into aerochamber.

     Emits spray that allows finer particles to be inhaled. Large droplets are retained in aerochamber.

   g. Breathe in slowly and fully.

     Ensures particles of medication are distributed to deeper airways.

   h. Hold full breath for 5-10 seconds.

     Ensures full drug distribution.

   i. Repeat for second puff.

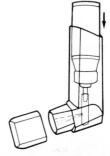

Fig. 75

Steps	Rationale
5. Instruct client to wait 5-10 minutes between inhalations or as ordered by physician.	Drugs must be inhaled sequentially. First inhalation opens airways and reduces inflammation. Second or third inhalations penetrate deeper airways.
6. Instruct client against repeating inhalations before next scheduled dose.	Drugs are prescribed at intervals during day to provide constant bronchodilation and minimize side effects.
7. Explain that client may feel gagging sensation in throat caused by droplets of medication on pharynx or tongue.	Results when inhalant is sprayed and inhaled incorrectly.
8. Instruct client in removing medication canister and cleaning inhaler in warm water.	Accumulation of spray around mouthpiece can interfere with proper distribution during use.
9. Ask if client has any questions.	Provides opportunity to clarify misconceptions or misunderstanding.
10. Ask client for any questions.	Provides opportunity to clarify misconceptions or misunderstandings.
11. Have client demonstrate use of inhaler.	Return demonstration provides feedback for measuring client's learning.
12. Record in nurse's notes content or skills taught and client's ability to use inhaler.	Provides continuity to teaching plan so other members of nursing staff will not teach same material.

Nurse Alert

Client may gag or swallow medication if unable to inhale while spray is administered. Client's need for bronchodilator more than every 4 hours can signal worsening of the respiratory conditions and the client's physician needs to be notified.

Clients who use steroid inhalers are at risk for topical *Candida* infection in the mouth and posterior pharynx. The nurse should observe for patchy white areas in the client's mouth.

Client Teaching

Instruct the client on proper use of an inhaler and the common side effects to expect. Explain the common signs and symptoms of xanthine and sympathomimetic drug overuse: tachycardia, palpitations, headache, restlessness, insomnia. Instruct the client to properly clean the inhaler to avoid transmission of microorganisms. Instruct client to inspect mouth daily for signs of *Candida* infection, patchy white lesions in mouth.

Pediatric Considerations

Children may not be able to learn how to use an inhaler until they reach school age. They also may need to pinch their nose shut during inhalation to gain the drug's effects.

Geriatric Considerations

Elderly clients with hand tremors or weakness in their ability to grasp objects may not be able to use an inhaler.

Instilling Vaginal Medication

Vaginal medications come in cream and suppository and are used to treat localized infection or inflammation. It is important to avoid embarrassing the client when administering these preparations. Often the client will prefer learning how to self-administer the medication. Because the discharge that is symptomatic of vaginal infections can be foul smelling, it is important to offer good perineal hygiene for the client.

Potential Nursing Diagnoses

Pain related to vaginal irritation
Body-image disturbance related to vaginal infection
Sexual dysfunction related to vaginal infection

Equipment

Medication ticket or form

Vaginal Suppository	Vaginal Cream
Suppository	Cream
Clean disposable gloves	Plastic applicator
Lubricating jelly	Clean disposable gloves
Clean tissues	Paper towel
Suppository inserter (optional)	Perineal pad (optional)
Perineal pad (optional)	

Steps	Rationale
1. Review physician's order for name of drug, dosage, and route of administration.	Ensures safe and accurate administration of drug.
2. Wash hands.	Reduces risk of transferring microorganisms.

Steps	Rationale
3. Explain procedure to client.	Reduces client anxiety.
4. Check client's identification band and ask client's name.	Ensures that right client receives right medication.
5. Have client lie in dorsal recumbent position.	Provides easy access to and good exposure of vaginal canal. Dependent position of client allows suppository to dissolve in vagina without escaping through orifice.
6. Keep abdomen and lower extremities draped.	Minimizes client embarrassment.
7. Apply disposable gloves.	Prevents transmission of infection between nurse and client.

Suppository

1. Remove suppository from foil wrapper and apply liberal amount of petrolatum jelly to smooth or rounded end. Lubricate gloved index finger of dominant hand.	Reduces friction against mucosal surfaces during insertion.
2. With nondominant gloved hand gently retract labial folds.	Exposes vaginal orifice.
3. Insert rounded end of suppository along posterior wall of vaginal canal length of index finger (7.5 to 10 cm [3 to 4 inches]). (Fig. 76)	Ensures equal distribution of medication along walls of vaginal cavity.
4. Withdraw finger and wipe away any remaining lubricant from around orifice and labia.	Maintains client comfort.
5. Remove gloves by pulling them inside out and discard them in appropriate receptacle.	Prevents spread of microorganisms.
6. Instruct client to remain on her back for at least 10 minutes.	Allows medication to melt and be absorbed into vaginal mucosa.

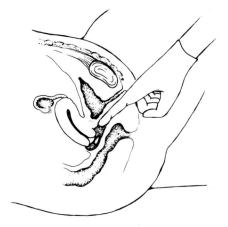

Fig. 76

Steps	Rationale
7. Offer perineal pad before client resumes ambulation.	Provides for client comfort.
8. Wash hands. NOTE: Follow same procedure when using suppository inserter.	Reduces transfer of microorganisms.
9. Record in medication record drug administered.	Prompt documentation prevents drug errors.

Vaginal Cream

1. Fill cream applicator, following package directions.	Dosage is prescribed by volume in applicator.
2. With your nondominant gloved hand, gently retract labial folds.	Exposes vaginal orifice.
3. With your dominant gloved hand, insert applicator approximately 7.5 cm (3 inches). Push applicator plunger to deposit medication.	Allows for equal distribution of medication along walls of vaginal cavity.
4. Withdraw plunger and place it on a paper towel. Wipe off any residual cream from labia or vaginal orifice.	Residual cream on applicator may contain microorganisms.

Steps	Rationale
5. Remove gloves and turn them inside out. Dispose of them in appropriate receptacle.	Disposing of gloves in this way reduces transfer of microorganisms.
6. Instruct client to remain flat on her back for at least 10 minutes.	Cream will be distributed and absorbed evenly in vaginal cavity rather than being lost through vaginal orifice.
7. Wash applicator with soap and warm water. Store it for future use.	Vaginal cavity is not sterile. Soap and water will assist in removing bacteria and residual cream.
8. Offer client a perineal pad before she resumes ambulation.	Provides client comfort.
9. Wash your hands.	Reduces transmission of microorganisms.
10. Record in medication record drug administered.	Prompt documentation prevents drug errors.

Nurse Alert

If suppository fails to dissolve and solid form is expelled, check expiration date on package.

Client Teaching

Clients often prefer to learn how to self-administer vaginal preparations. Using a step-by-step approach, allow the client to do a demonstration of the technique. It is important that she insert the suppository or cream correctly into the vaginal canal.

Geriatric Considerations

An elderly woman may have difficulty assuming a position that allows for self-administration of vaginal preparations. Arthritic conditions of the hips, knees, or upper extremities can make self-administration painful and difficult.

Inserting a Rectal Suppository

There are various types of drugs available in suppository form that create local as well as systemic effects. Aminophylline suppositories act systemically to dilate the respiratory bronchioles. A Dulcolax suppository acts locally to promote defecation. Suppositories are safe to administer. The nurse should be concerned primarily with placing the suppository correctly against the rectal mucosal wall, past the internal anal sphincter, so the suppository will not be expelled. Clients who have had rectal surgery or are experiencing rectal bleeding should not be given a suppository.

Potential Nursing Diagnoses

Alteration in health maintenance related to mobility restriction (client unable to self-administer drug)
Knowledge deficit regarding drug therapy
Constipation

Equipment

Medication ticket or form
Rectal suppository
Lubricating jelly
Clean disposable gloves
Tissue

Steps	Rationale
1. Review physician's order for name of drug, dosage, and route of administration.	Ensures that drug will be administered safely and accurately.
2. Wash hands.	Reduces transfer of microorganisms.
3. Explain procedure to client.	Reduces client anxiety.

Steps	Rationale
4. Check client's identification band and ask client's name.	Ensures that right client receives right medication.
5. Ask client to assume a side-lying (Sims) position with upper leg flexed upward.	Exposes anus and helps client relax external anal sphincter.
6. Keep client draped with only anal area exposed.	Draping client maintains privacy and facilitates relaxation.
7. Remove suppository from its foil wrapper and lubricate rounded end with jelly. Lubricate gloved index finger of your dominant hand.	Lubrication reduces friction as suppository enters rectum.
8. Ask client to take slow deep breaths through his mouth and to relax anal sphincter.	Forcing suppository through a constricted sphincter causes pain.
9. Retract client's buttocks with your nondominant hand. With your gloved index finger, insert suppository gently through anus, past internal anal sphincter, and against rectal wall: 10 cm (4 inches) in adults, 5 cm (2 inches) in children and infants. (Fig. 77)	Suppository must be placed against rectal mucosa for eventual absorption and therapeutic action.
10. Withdraw your finger and wipe off client's anal area.	Provides client comfort.

Fig. 77

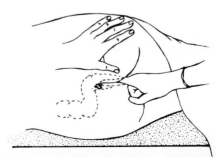

Steps	Rationale
11. Discard gloves by turning them inside out and dispose of them in appropriate receptacle.	Disposing of gloves in this way reduces transfer of microorganisms.
12. Instruct client to remain flat or on his side for 5 minutes.	Prevents expulsion of the suppository.
13. If suppository contains a laxative or fecal softener, place call light within client's reach so he can obtain assistance to reach a bedpan or toilet.	Being able to call for assistance provides client with sense of control over elimination.
14. Wash your hands.	Reduces transfer of microorganisms.
15. Record in medication record drug administered.	Prompt documentation prevents drug errors.

Nurse Alert

Although it is unusual, a client may experience a vagal reflex response (slowing of the heart rate) as a result of excessive rectal stimulation.

Client Teaching

Clients may prefer learning how to self-administer rectal suppositories. This can be difficult unless the nurse is clear as to how to insert the suppository past the internal anal sphincter. A client must be familiar with the sensation felt as the sphincter relaxes over the insertion finger.

Pediatric Considerations

The rectal route is chosen only when children are unable to take food or liquid by mouth and when it is unlikely that they have large amounts of stool. The rectum must be empty for effective drug absorption.

Geriatric Considerations

An elderly client may have mobility restrictions that prohibit self-administration of suppositories.

INFECTION
CONTROL

Handwashing

Nosocomial infections are infections that result from the delivery of health services in a health care facility. They are associated with diagnostic or therapeutic procedures and often involve extended stays, thus increasing the cost of health care to both the client and the health care worker.

The use of masks, protective eyewear, gloves, and specialized gowns assists in reducing the risk of transmission of blood-borne pathogens (CDC, 1988; Pugliese and Lampinen, 1989). Along with these aids to infection control, the nurse must remember that handwashing is the most important and basic technique in preventing and controlling infection (CDC, 1988). However, the ideal duration of handwashing is not known. The Centers for Disease Control (CDC) and Public Health Service note that washing times of at least 10 to 15 seconds will remove most transient microorganisms from the skin (Garner and Favero, 1985). If hands are visibly soiled, more time may be needed. Agency policies often recommend staff to wash hands for 1 to 2 minutes after working in high-risk areas (e.g., trauma units, emergency rooms, etc.). Routine handwashing may be performed with bar, liquid, or granule soap, or soap-impregnated tissue.

Potential Nursing Diagnoses

Potential for infection

Equipment

Sink with warm running water
Soap or disinfectant in foot-operated dispenser (or bar soap)
Paper towels
Orange stick (optional)

Steps	Rationale
1. Push wristwatch and long uniform sleeves up above your wrists. Remove jewelry.	Provides complete access to fingers, hands, and wrists. Jewelry may harbor microorganisms.
2. Keep your fingernails short and filed.	Dirt and secretions that lodge under the fingernails contain microorganisms. Long fingernails can scratch client's skin.
3. Inspect surface of your hands and fingers for any breaks or cuts in skin and cuticles. Report such lesions when caring for highly susceptible clients.	Open cuts or wounds can harbor high concentrations of microorganisms. Such lesions may serve as portals of exit, increasing client's exposure to infection, or as portals of entry, increasing your risk of acquiring an infection.
4. Stand in front of sink, keeping hands and uniform away from sink surface. (If hands touch sink during handwashing, repeat the process.) Use a sink where it is comfortable to reach faucet.	Inside of sink is a contaminated area. Reaching over sink increases risk of touching edge, which is contaminated.
5. Turn on water. Press foot pedals with foot to regulate flow and temperature. Push knee pedals laterally to control flow and temperature. Turn on handoperated faucets by covering faucet with paper towel.	When hands come in contact with faucet, they are considered contaminated. Organisms spread easily from hands to faucet.
6. Avoid splashing water against your uniform.	Microorganisms travel and grow in moisture.
7. Regulate flow of water so temperature is warm.	Warm water is more comfortable. Hot water opens pores of skin, causing irritation.

Steps	Rationale
8. Wet hands and lower arms thoroughly under running water. Keep hands and forearms lower than elbows during washing. (Fig. 78)	Hands are the most contaminated parts to be washed. Water flows from least to most contaminated area.
9. Apply 1 ml of regular or 3 ml of antiseptic liquid soap to hands and lather thoroughly. If bar soap is used, hold it throughout the lathering period. Soap granules and leaflet preparations may be used.	Bar soap should be rinsed before return to soap dish. A soap dish that allows water to drain keeps soap firm. Jelly-like soap permits growth of microorganisms.
10. Wash hands using plenty of lather and friction for 15-30 seconds. Interlace fingers and rub palms and back of hands with circular motion. (Fig. 79)	Soap cleanses by emulsifying fat and oil and lowering surface tension. Friction and rubbing mechanically loosen and remove dirt and transient bacteria. Interlacing fingers and thumbs ensures that all surfaces are cleansed.
11. If areas underlying fingernails are soiled, clean them with fingernails of other hand and additional soap or a clean orangewood stick. Do not tear or cut skin under or around nail.	Mechanical removal of dirt and sediment under nails reduces microorganisms on hands.
12. Rinse hands and wrists thoroughly, keeping hands down and elbows up.	Rinsing mechanically washes away dirt and microorganisms.

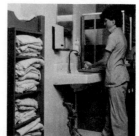

Fig. 78

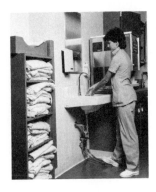

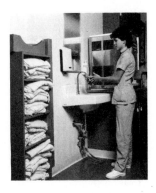

Fig. 79   Fig. 80

Steps	Rationale
13. Repeat Steps 9 through 11 but extend actual period of washing for 1-, 2-, and 3-minute handwashings.	Greater the likelihood that hands will be contaminated, greater the need for thorough handwashing.
14. Dry hands thoroughly, wiping from fingers down to wrists and forearms. (Fig. 80)	Dry from cleanest area (fingertips) to least clean (wrists) to avoid contamination. Drying hands prevents chapping and roughened skin.
15. Discard paper towel in proper receptacle.	Proper disposal of contaminated objects prevents transfer of microorganisms.
16. Turn off water with foot and knee pedals. To turn off a hand faucet, use a clean dry paper towel.	Wet towel and wet hands allow transfer of pathogens by capillary action.
17. Keep hands and cuticles well lubricated with hand lotion or moisturizer between washings.	Dry chapped skin cracks easily, creating portal of entry for infection.

Nurse Alert

If the nurse has an open lesion or wound on her hand, some agencies have policies prohibiting her contact with clients.

Care of a Client in Isolation

The nurse must follow special precautions when caring for clients who either have greater susceptibility to infection or are carriers of microorganisms that can be easily transmitted to other persons. Protective isolation or isolation precautions keep the affected client within the confines of his room. The nurse uses protective coverings such as a mask, gown, or gloves depending on how the organism is transmitted and how susceptible the client is to infection. Staying within a confined area and being cared for by nurses covered in protective clothing are factors that can cause a person to feel socially isolated. Whenever the nurse cares for the client in isolation, it is important to maintain therapeutic communication and provide a personalized approach to care.

Potential Nursing Diagnoses

Potential for infection related to decreased immunity
Sensory alteration related to isolation

Equipment

The selection of equipment depends on the type of care to be administered to the client (for example, supplies for administering medications, supplies for hygiene, supplies for bedmaking).

Steps	Rationale
1. Refer to physician's orders for type of isolation in which client is to be placed.	Type of isolation category influences type of protective clothing worn and precautions followed.
2. Refer to policy and procedure manual or infection control policy of institution for precautions to follow.	Each institution may require guidelines that vary from CDC recommendations.

Steps	Rationale
3. Review laboratory test results to determine type of microorganisms for which client is being isolated.	Allows you to know what microorganism is infecting client and medium in which it was identified (e.g., sputum, blood, wound). This information will enable you to be appropriately cautious when handling infected exudate or drainage.
4. Consider types of care measures or procedures to be performed while in client's room.	Helps you anticipate needs for supplies, time your organization while in room, and coordinate your activities.
5. Prepare all necessary equipment and supplies.	Prevents need to leave and reenter room several times, increasing risk of infection.

Donning Protective Clothing

1. Wash hands.	Reduces transmission of microorganisms.
2. Remove gown from cart. Grasp top of gown at inside with outside facing away from you and allow gown to unfold. (Fig. 81)	Opens gown fully for easier application. Clean gown is not sterile, so you may touch all sides. If gown is reused, outer surface is considered contaminated.
3. Slide your arms forward through sleeves until cuffs cover your wrists. (Fig. 82)	Gown should have long sleeves with tight-fitting cuffs to provide full protection.

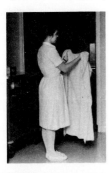
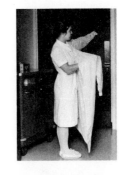

Fig. 81   Fig. 82

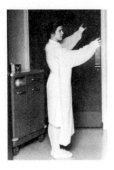

Fig. 83

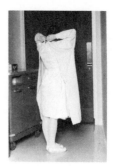

Fig. 84

Steps	Rationale
4. Pull gown onto and around your shoulders. (Fig. 83)	Gown should completely cover your uniform.
5. Secure ties at neck. (Fig. 84)	Keeps gown in place.
6. Secure ties at your waist.	Prevents gown from falling away from your body, which can cause contamination of your uniform.
7. Put on clean disposable gloves, being sure that edge of glove covers cuff of gown.	Prevents transmission of pathogens by direct and indirect contact.
8. Apply mask securely over your face and mouth (see Skill 6-4).	Protects you from inhaling large-particle aerosols and small-particle droplets. Also protects susceptible clients from organisms that you might spread.

Preparing to Enter Room

1. Leave medication cart or tray outside client's room.	Prevents contamination from repeated transfer in and out of room.
2. Leave brown paper bag and isolation label for specimen collection on isolation cart.	Specimen will eventually be placed in bag, so outer surface of bag remains clean. Thus anyone can transport specimen without fear of contamination.

Steps	Rationale
3. Place stethoscope on inside handle of door or on paper towel away from bedside work area.	Stethoscope should remain free of contamination as you perform care.
4. Avoid taking into room any equipment or supplies that are absolutely essential for use with other clients or by other personnel.	Exposure of equipment to infected material results in contamination. Equipment must be disinfected or sterilized before reuse.

Entering Room

1. Take all necessary equipment and supplies into room. Avoid placing on contaminated surfaces.	Minimizes transmission of microorganisms.
2. Lower glove cuff, remove watch, and place on clean paper towel within easy view.	Wristwatch is used for vital sign measurement and should remain uncontaminated since it is later removed from room.
3. Place specimen containers on clean paper towel in client's bathroom.	Specimen containers will be handled by laboratory personnel. Contamination should be kept to minimum. Urine and feces should be transferred in bathroom.

Vital Signs

1. Take stethoscope and place it around neck. During use, be sure that it has minimal contact with contaminated material (e.g., drainage, excretions).	Stethoscope will be reused with other clients and should not contact contaminated material.
2. Measure client's temperature using proper technique (Skills 2-1 to 2-4).	
3. Measure client's blood pressure (Skill 2-8). (Wrap cuff around thin gown sleeve, above antecubital fossa.)	Minimizes contamination of cuff.

Steps	Rationale
4. With watch in view on towel, assess pulse and respirations (Skills 2-5 through 2-7).	If gloved hand touches client or any contaminated object, watch should not be touched.
5. Record results of vital signs on clean paper towel at bedside.	Chart and flow sheets cannot be taken into client's room. You will transcribe results onto form outside room once all care is completed.
6. Place stethoscope on clean surface in room. Wash off diaphragm or bell, if soiled, with alcohol swab.	Stethoscope will be removed from room when nursing care is completed. Alcohol helps disinfect soiled surfaces.

Medications

1. Administer medications using appropriate technique (Unit V).	
2. After administering injection, discard contaminated needle and syringe in appropriate containers (e.g., needle cutter) in client's room. Dispose of cups and wrappers in container in room.	Prevents exposure of personnel to contaminated objects by avoiding transport of equipment to medication room.

Specimen Collection

1. Collect necessary specimens using appropriate technique. Transfer specimen to container by minimizing contact of gloved hands with outer surface of container.	Each type of body excretion or exudate must be collected in specific manner to prevent contamination by resident flora. Containers will be handled by laboratory personnel and should remain clean on outside.
2. Be sure that specimen container is sealed tightly.	Prevents spillage and contamination of its outer surface.
3. Label specimen container with client's name.	Properly labeled specimens are essential so correct laboratory results are reported for correct client.

Steps	Rationale
4. Have nurse stand outside client's room holding brown paper bag. Place specimen in bag without contaminating bag's outer surface.	Outer surface of bag is considered clean and can be touched by personnel.
5. Ask second nurse to place isolation label on bag and have specimen transported.	Specimens should be transported to laboratory immediately for proper preparation.

Hygiene (Unit VII)

1. Perform necessary hygiene measures. Avoid allowing gown to become wet.	Moisture on gown provides path for microorganisms to spread to your uniform.
2. Discard soiled linen into special isolation linen bag located in client's room.	Isolation linen bag must be impervious and sturdy to contain contaminated linen.

Bagging Articles

1. If linen bag is filled, be sure that all soiled linen is contained and that top of bag is securely tied. (Fig. 85)	Contaminated linen should be well contained to prevent exposure to health care personnel.
2. Have second nurse stand outside client's room and hold clean linen bag. (Fig. 86)	Double bagging prevents exposure of personnel to contaminated outer surface of soiled linen bag.

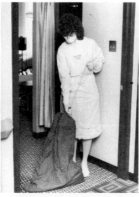

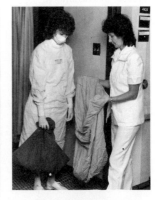

Fig. 85   Fig. 86

Steps	Rationale
3. Nurse outside room holds clean bag by folding its top edges back to form a cuff over her hands.	Cuff protects you from contacting soiled linen bag.
4. As opening of bag separates, place your hand inside clean bag and pull opening out fully.	Inside of bag is considered contaminated. Outer bag should be opened so contaminated bag can be easily dropped in.
5. Drop contaminated linen bag into clean receiving bag without touching receiving bag's sides. (Fig. 87)	Contaminated bag is contained and can now be transported outside client's room.
6. Have second nurse discard linen into appropriate hamper.	Institutional policy may vary as to where to dispose of isolation linen.
7. Take any contaminated reusable objects (e.g., suction bottles or instruments) and carefully place in paper or plastic bag held by second nurse outside room.	CDC recommends single bag as adequate to discard items if bag impervious and sturdy and article can be placed inside it without contaminating outer surface. Otherwise, follow double-bag procedure.
8. Second nurse seals bag with tape or according to agency policy.	Contains contaminated item safely.

Preparing to Leave Room

1. Be sure that client's needs have been attended to.	Attempt to minimize number of visits into isolation room, particularly when strict precautions are being followed. You may not return to room for some time.

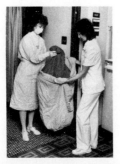

Fig. 87

Steps	Rationale
2. Remove gloves by grasping cuff of one glove and pulling it off, turning glove inside out. With your ungloved hand, tuck finger inside cuff of remaining glove and pull off, turning inside out. Dispose of it in proper receptacle.	Gloves are removed first since they are most likely to be contaminated and should not be used to touch hair around mask.
3. Untie or pull off mask from around your ears and dispose of it in receptacle.	Masks are disposable.
4. Untie gown from around your neck and waist. Keeping your hand inside one cuff, pull opposite sleeve down from arm. Do same for other arm.	Keeping hands inside gown minimizes contact with microorganisms.
5. Pull gown off by turning it inside out. Fold so contaminated sides face one another. Discard in proper receptacle.	Gown is turned inside out so hands and clothing do not come in contact with contaminated outer surface.
6. Wash your hands thoroughly.	Mechanically removes any transient microorganisms contacted.
7. Pick up wristwatch and stethoscope, taking care not to touch a contaminated surface. Note vital sign recordings made in room.	Clean hands may touch watch and stethoscope.
8. Leave room, closing door securely.	Room should remain closed, especially when airborne infection is being isolated.
9. Record in nurse's notes vital signs and other procedures according to guidelines for each skill.	Documents care provided.

Nurse Alert

Be sure that you are familiar with the specific guidelines for each isolation category. It is important to know what type of infection the client has and in what manner the infective organisms are transmitted.

Client Teaching

Explain the purpose for and importance of isolation techniques. Clients must understand that the precautions used are for everyone's safety. If the client understands isolation practices, he can help enforce procedures when visitors enter the room.

Pediatric Considerations

Preschoolers may view isolation as a form of punishment. Older children should be given a thorough explanation of procedures to minimize fears and fantasies. Show children the different forms of protective clothing. Young children can play "dress up" with masks and gloves. If possible, allow children to see your face before applying a mask.

Geriatric Considerations

Elderly clients may be more at risk than younger clients of sensory deprivation due to normal aging processes. They will consistently need meaningful sensory stimuli while in isolation. Some simple actions to take might include turning on the lights when entering the room, raising the head of the bed and repositioning the client, opening window shades or curtains, and sitting down to have a relaxed discussion.

Protective Eyewear

The use of protective eyewear, either goggles or face shield, is to prevent the transmission of pathogens by way of the health care worker's mucous membranes (e.g., around the eye, nasal, and oral cavities). This protection is recommended when health care workers are in areas where suctioning, dressing changes, or hygiene care can cause the splattering of blood and/or body fluids on the health care worker (Pugliese and Lampinen, 1989).

Potential Nursing Diagnoses

Potential for infection related to droplet contamination

Equipment

Plastic face shield
    or
Plastic eye goggles

Steps	Rationale
1. Wash hands.	Reduces transmission of micro-organisms.
2. Apply protective eyewear.	

Goggles

Secure goggles comfortably over eyes. Tighten as needed.	Goggles reduce the risk of blood/body fluid droplet transmission to the mucous membranes of the eyes only.

Steps	Rationale

Face Shield

Secure shield over top of the head. Move shield over the face and adjust as needed to protect the worker's facial mucous membranes.

Face shields offer more protection to the mucous membranes of the face. During procedures resulting in a splattering of droplets of blood and body fluids, this type of protection is recommended.

3. After procedure is completed, either leave protective goggles or shield at the client's bedside or discard in appropriate receptacle.
Do not wear goggles or shield outside the client's room.

Protective shields may be worn more than once for nonsterile procedures.
Proper disposal reduces transmission of pathogens.
Wearing protective eye shields in the hall, etc., increases risk of transmission of pathogens.

4. Wash hands.

Reduces transmission of microorganisms.

Nurse Alert

These protective devices are designed to reduce the risk of transmission of blood-borne pathogens to the nurse. These are not ordered by the physicians. It is a nursing judgment to wear these shields. In certain agencies the wearing of these face protectors is mandatory in high-risk situations (e.g., trauma units, care of AIDS client with a respiratory infection, operating rooms).

Donning a Surgical
Mask

A mask may be worn for several reasons: as a precaution to reduce air-droplet transmission of microorganisms while caring for
a client in isolation, when assisting with a sterile procedure, or
when preparing sterile supplies for a sterile field. The nurse
should apply the mask snugly around face and nose; otherwise it
is ineffective in controlling air-droplet nuclei. A mask is always
applied before the nurse performs a surgical handwash. When a
mask becomes moist, it should be changed. Moisture promotes
the spread of microorganisms.

Potential Nursing Diagnoses

Potential for infection related to droplet contamination

Equipment

Clean disposable mask

Steps	Rationale
Application of Mask	
1. Find top edge of mask (usually has a thin metal strip along edge).	Pliable metal fits snugly against bridge of nose.
2. Hold mask by top two strings or loops. Tie two top ties at the top of the back of your head, with ties *above* your ears (alternative: slip loops over each ear). (Fig. 88)	Position of ties at top of head provides tight fit. Ties over ears may cause irritation.
3. Tie two lower ties snugly around your neck, with mask well under chin. (Fig. 89)	Prevents escape of microorganisms through sides of mask as you talk or breathe.

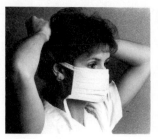

Fig. 88

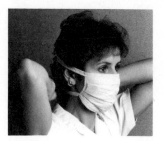

Fig. 89

Steps	Rationale
4. Gently pinch upper metal band around the bridge of your nose.	Prevents microorganisms from escaping around nose.

Removal of Mask

1. If you have gloves on, remove them and wash your hands.	Prevents contamination of hair, neck, and face from contact with soiled gloves.
2. Untie both ties and fold mask in half with inner surfaces together.	Avoids contact with contaminated inner surface.
3. Dispose of mask in receptacle.	Reduces spread of infection.

Nurse Alert

In the operating room, apply a second mask over the first once the first mask becomes moist. Removal of a mask in the surgical area causes immediate contamination of surrounding objects.

Client Teaching

When caring for a client in isolation, explain the purpose of a mask. The mask may add to a client's feeling of becoming depersonalized.

Pediatric Considerations

If a child is awake in the operating room, allow him to see your face, if possible, before applying the mask.

Surgical Handwashing

Nurses who work in sterile areas such as the operating room or labor and delivery rooms must practice surgical handwashing. The technique requires greater effort than routine handwashing. During a surgical scrub the nurse washes a wider area, from fingertips to elbows. Usually the duration of a scrub lasts 5 to 10 minutes to ensure that all skin surfaces are thoroughly cleaned. For maximal cleansing and removal of bacteria the nurse removes all jewelry from her fingers and arms and keeps her fingernails short, clean, and free of polish.

Potential Nursing Diagnoses

Potential for infection related to transient skin bacteria

Equipment

Deep sink with foot pedals or knee controls
Antiseptic detergent in a foot-controlled dispenser
Hand brushes
Orange stick or disposable nail file

Steps	Rationale
1. Check hands and fingers for cuts or abrasions	Areas of inflammation or breaks in skin can harbor microorganisms.
2. Remove all jewelry.	Harbors microorganisms.
3. Apply a face mask, making certain to cover your nose and mouth snugly.	Prevents escape of microorganisms into air, which can contaminate hands.
4. Adjust water flow to lukewarm temperature.	Hot water removes protective oils from the skin and increases skin's sensitivity to soap.

Steps	Rationale
5. Wet your hands and forearms liberally, keeping hands above level of elbows during entire procedure. NOTE: Your scrub dress or uniform must be kept dry.	Water runs by gravity from fingertips to elbows. Hands become cleanest part of upper extremity. Keeping hands elevated allows water to flow from least to most contaminated area.
6. Dispense a liberal amount of soap (2-5 ml) into hands and lather hands and arms to 5 cm (2 inches) above elbows.	Washing wide area reduces risk of contaminating overlying gown that you will apply.
7. Clean nails with orange stick or file under running water. (Fig. 90)	Removes dirt and organic material that harbor large numbers of microorganisms.
8. Rinse hands and arms thoroughly, keeping your hands above level of elbows.	Removes transient bacteria from fingers, hands, and forearms.
9. Lather your hands and arms and scrub each hand with brush for 45 seconds. Using same brush, scrub each arm to 5 cm (2 inches) above elbow. Divide arm into thirds: scrub each lower forearm 15 seconds, each upper forearm 15 seconds, and 5 cm above each elbow 15 seconds. (Fig. 91)	Scrubbing loosens resident bacteria that adhere to skin's surface.

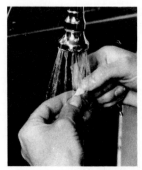

Fig. 90

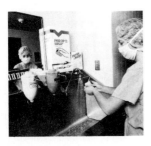

Fig. 91

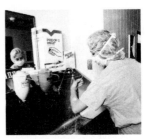

Fig. 92

Steps	Rationale
10. Discard brush and rinse your hands and arms thoroughly.	After touching skin, brush is considered contaminated. Rinsing removes resident bacteria.
11. Using second brush, scrub each hand for 30 seconds. Use same brush to scrub each arm up to elbow. Divide arm in half: scrub each lower forearm 15 seconds and each upper forearm 15 seconds.	Second scrubbing ensures thorough cleaning of hands and forearms. Number of resident microorganisms remaining on skin will be minimal.
12. Discard brush and rinse your hands and arms thoroughly. Turn off water with foot pedal. (Fig. 92)	Prevents contamination of hands.
13. Use sterile towel to dry one hand thoroughly, moving from fingers to elbow. Dry in a rotating motion. NOTE: If you wish to apply sterile gloves for use in a regular clinical area you need not use brushes or dry your hands with sterile towels. Thorough lathering and friction performed twice according to procedure will ensure clean hands. In this situation you may use clean paper towels for drying.	Dry from cleanest to least clean area. Drying prevents chapping and facilitates donning of gloves.

Steps	Rationale
14. Repeat drying method for other hand, using different area of towel or a new sterile towel.	Prevents contamination of hand.
15. Keep hands higher than elbows and away from your body.	Prevents accidental contamination.
16. Proceed into operating room or labor and delivery area, keeping hands from contacting any object.	If your hands touch any object, scrub must be repeated.

Nurse Alert

Throughout the procedure and afterwards the nurse must not allow an unsterile object to touch her hands or lower arms.

Donning a Sterile Gown

The nurse must wear a sterile gown in the operating room and delivery room so sterile objects can be comfortably handled with less risk of contamination. Nurses assisting physicians with invasive procedures in a treatment room may also wear sterile gowns. A gown is applied after surgical handwashing and after the nurse has donned a mask and surgical cap. She either picks up the gown from a sterile field or has a gowned assistant hand her one.

The entire surface of the gown is not considered sterile. Only the area from the anterior waist to, but not including, the collar and anterior surface of the sleeves is sterile.

Potential Nursing Diagnoses

This procedure may be performed by nurses caring for clients with a variety of nursing diagnoses.

Equipment

Disposable mask
Disposable cap
Sterile gown (prepared for donning by circulating nurse)

Steps	Rationale
1. Don mask and cap. Carry out surgical handscrubbing for at least 5 minutes (Skill 6-5).	Scrubbing eliminates microorganisms from surface of hands. Mask and cap reduce chances of transmitting organisms to gown by direct contact and airborne transmission.
2. Pick up gown, grasping inside surface at collar. (Fig. 93)	Hands are not completely sterile. Inside surface of gown will contact skin surface and is thus considered contaminated.

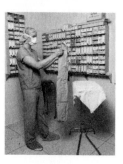 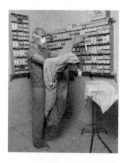

Fig. 93   Fig. 94

Steps	Rationale
3. Stand away from sterile pack and table. Hold gown at arm's length away from your body and allow gown to unfold by itself. Be careful not to allow gown to touch floor. (Fig. 93)	Contact of outer surface of gown with a dirty or clean surface would result in gown contamination. Shaking of gown can cause air currents that increase risk of contamination.
4. Hold gown by inside, open shoulder seams, and insert each hand through armholes. (Fig. 94)	Inside surface of gown is considered contaminated.
5. Keeping your upper arms in front of you at shoulder height, extend hands toward gown cuff. (Do not push hands through cuffs if using closed glove method.)	Extension of arms straight ahead keeps sterile outer surface of gown in view and reduces risk of touching floor or a portion of your body.
6. Have circulating nurse assist by reaching inside gown and pulling inner shoulder and side seams onto your shoulders.	Working from behind scrub nurse prevents contamination by circulating nurse. Gown should fit comfortably.
7. Have circulating nurse tie or snap gown at neckline and waist. Only ties or snaps should be touched. (Fig. 95)	Provides secure fit without contamination.

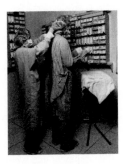

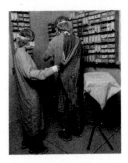

Fig. 95

Fig. 96

Steps	Rationale
8. If gown is a wraparound style, enclose waist tie or snap in front with a sterile towel. (Keep your hands inside sleeves while grasping towel.) Hand sterile towel to circulating nurse.	Towel provides a surface that circulating nurse can grasp without contaminating gown.
9. Circulating nurse grasps edge of towel without touching tie while you pivot in opposite direction from her. (Fig. 96)	Wraparound gown achieves better coverage of your body and reduces risk of contamination.
10. Take tie from towel wrapper, keeping your hands inside sleeves, and tie gown in front. Make certain that gown is completely closed.	Gown must be securely tied while worn in operating room.

Nurse Alert

If the gown comes in contact with any unsterile object, including the nurse's hands, it is considered to be contaminated.

Open Gloving

The nurse applies sterile gloves by the open method when preparing to work with certain types of sterile equipment and when performing sterile procedures such as dressing changes or catheter insertion. The gloves provide a barrier between the nurse's hands and the objects she contacts. She is able to freely touch objects in a sterile field without concern of contamination. When wearing sterile gloves, she should always remain conscious of which objects are sterile and which are not. A glove becomes contaminated whenever it contacts a nonsterile object.

Potential Nursing Diagnoses

This procedure may be performed by nurses caring for clients with a variety of nursing diagnoses.

Equipment

Package of sterile gloves of proper size

Steps	Rationale
1. Wash hands thoroughly.	Reduces numbers of microorganisms residing on surfaces of hands.
2. Remove outer package wrapper by carefully peeling apart sides.	Prevents inner glove package from accidentally opening and touching contaminated objects.
3. Grasp inner package and lay it on a clean flat surface just above waist level. Open package, keeping gloves on wrapper's inside surface.	Sterile object held below your waist is considered contaminated. Inner surface of glove package is considered sterile.

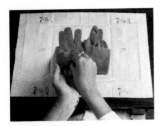

Fig. 97

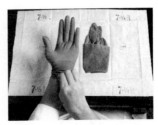

Fig. 98

Steps	Rationale
4. If gloves are not prepowdered, take packet of powder and apply lightly to hands over a sink or wastebasket.	Powder allows gloves to slip on easily. (Some physicians do not use powder for fear of promoting growth of microorganisms).
5. Identify right and left glove. Each glove has a cuff approximately 5 cm (2 inches) wide. Glove your dominant hand first.	Proper identification of gloves prevents contamination by improper fit. Gloving of dominant hand first improves your dexterity with procedure.
6. With thumb and first two fingers of your nondominant hand, grasp edge of cuff of glove for dominant hand. Touch only the glove's inside surface. (Fig. 97)	Inner edge of cuff will lie against your skin and thus is not considered sterile. NOTE: Left hand dominant in photo.
7. Carefully pull glove over your dominant hand, leaving a cuff and being sure that cuff does not roll up your wrist. Be sure also that thumb and fingers are in proper spaces. (Fig. 98)	If glove's outer surface touches your hand or wrist, it is contaminated.
8. With your gloved dominant hand, slip your fingers underneath second glove's cuff. (Fig. 99)	Cuff protects your gloved fingers. Sterile touching sterile prevents glove contamination.

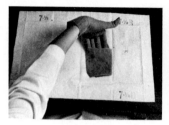

Fig. 99

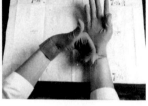

Fig. 100

Steps	Rationale
9. Carefully pull second glove over your nondominant hand. Do not allow fingers and thumb of gloved dominant hand to touch any part of your exposed nondominant hand. Keep thumb of dominant hand abducted back. (Fig. 100)	Contact of gloved hand with exposed hand results in contamination.
10. Once second glove is on, interlock your hands. Cuffs usually fall down after application. Be sure to touch only sterile sides. (Fig. 101)	Ensures smooth fit over fingers.

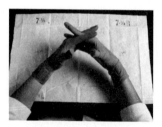

Fig. 101

Nurse Alert

If the outer (clean) surface of a glove touches a nonsterile object, such as a portion of your arm or the table surface, remove and repeat gloving.

Client Teaching

Explain to the client why gloves are used during a procedure. At times the client may perceive the use of gloves as the nurse's reluctance to touch him.

Closed Gloving

The technique of closed gloving is used primarily by nurses who work in sterile treatment areas such as the operating room or labor and delivery rooms. Closed gloving differs from open gloving in that the nurse's hands are kept covered by a sterile gown cuff throughout the procedure. Placement of each glove over a gown cuff provides added protection against contamination.

Potential Nursing Diagnoses

This procedure may be performed by nurses caring for clients with a variety of nursing diagnoses.

Equipment

Package of sterile gloves of correct size

Steps	Rationale
1. Don a sterile gown (according to Skill 6-6) after thorough handwashing.	Closed gloving is performed only after a sterile gown has been put on.
2. Have circulating nurse open glove package.	You can then easily pick up and apply gloves. Remember, you will be wearing sterile gown and cannot prepare gloves without contaminating gown.
3. Keep your scrubbed hands within sleeve of surgical gown at point of cuff seams.	Prevents your bare hands from contacting sterile exterior of gown.

Steps	Rationale

4. Grasp inside of cuff sleeve covering your nondominant hand. With same hand, pick up glove for your dominant hand. Place glove palm side down on palm of covered dominant hand. Have glove fingers pointing toward elbow of dominant arm. (Fig. 102)

Gown protects your fingers. Sterile touching sterile is sterile. Positioning of glove will allow you to slip it over gown cuff.

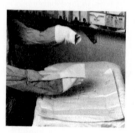

Fig. 102

5. Fingers of your covered dominant hand pinch underside of glove's cuff. With your covered nondominant hand, grasp topside of glove's cuff for dominant hand. Pull glove over gown cuff and fingers of dominant hand simultaneously. (Fig. 103)

Since your fingers do not exit through gown's cuff, gown and glove contamination is prevented.

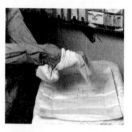

Fig. 103

6. Carefully push your fingers into glove and be sure glove's cuff covers gown's cuff.

Ensures proper fit. Glove fits over gown cuff to provide extra protection against contamination.

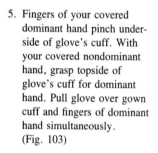

Steps	Rationale

7. With your gloved dominant hand, place opposite glove palm side down over palm of your covered nondominant hand, glove fingers toward elbow. (Fig. 104)

Sterile touching sterile is sterile.

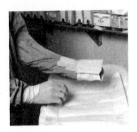

Fig. 104

8. Repeat Steps 5 and 6 for nondominant hand. (Figs. 105, 106)

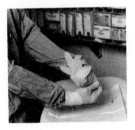

Fig. 105

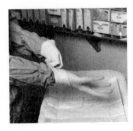

Fig. 106

9. Interlock gloved hands.

Ensures smooth fit over fingers.

Nurse Alert

If the glove contacts any nonsterile object, it is considered contaminated and the procedure must be repeated.

Tepid Sponging

A common form of therapeutic bath is tepid sponging. The procedure promotes the controlled loss of body heat through evaporation and conduction when clients have seriously elevated fevers. Since cooling occurs slowly, temperature fluctuations are avoided. The use of tepid water prevents chilling, which can cause an elevation in body temperature from muscular shivering.

Parents of small children learn how to safely administer tepid sponge baths in the home setting. Young children are at risk of having a seizure when fevers become high. The nurse in a health care setting can begin tepid sponging while pursuing additional orders from a physician for temperature control.

Potential Nursing Diagnoses

Hyperthermia related to infectious process
Knowledge deficit regarding fever management

Equipment

Bath basin	Waterproof pads
Tepid water (37° C [98.6° F])	Bath blanket
Bath thermometer	Ethyl alcohol (optional)
Washcloths	Thermometer

Steps	Rationale
1. Wash hands.	Reduces transmission of micro-organisms.
2. Explain to client that purpose of tepid sponging is to cool body slowly. Describe in brief the steps of procedure.	Procedure can be uncomfortable because of cool water application. Anxiety over procedure can increase body temperature.

Steps	Rationale
3. Close room curtain or door.	Maintains client privacy.
4. Measure client's temperature and pulse.	Provides baseline to measure effects of sponging.
5. Place waterproof pads under client and remove gown.	Pads prevent soiling of bed linen. Removing gown provides access to all skin surfaces.
6. Keep bath blanket over body parts not being sponged. Close windows and door to prevent drafts in room.	Bath blanket prevents chilling.
7. Check water temperature. Add equal parts ethyl alcohol and water (optional).	Alcohol evaporates at low body temperature to increase heat loss.
8. Immerse washcloths in water and apply wet cloths under each axilla and over groin. If using tub, immerse client 20-30 minutes.	Axilla and groin are areas containing large superficial blood vessels. Application of sponges promotes cooler temperature of the body's core by conduction. Immersion provides more effective heat loss.
9. Gently sponge an extremity for 5 min. Note client's response. Opposite extremity may be covered by a cool washcloth.	Prevents sudden temperature fall and minimizes risk of developing chills.
10. Dry extremity and reassess client's pulse and body temperature. Observe client's response to therapy.	Client's response to therapy is monitored to prevent sudden temperature change.
11. Continue sponging other extremities, back, and buttocks for 3-5 min each. Reassess temperature and pulse every 15 min.	Exposure of all body parts to sponging facilitates drop in body temperature.
12. Change water and reapply sponges to axilla and groin as needed.	Water temperature rises as result of exposure to client's warm body surface.

Steps	Rationale
13. When body temperature falls to slightly above normal (38° C or 100° F), discontinue procedure.	This prevents a temperature drift to a subnormal level.
14. Dry extremities and body parts thoroughly. Cover client with a light bath blanket or sheet.	Drying and covering client prevent chilling. Excessively heavy covering may increase body temperature.
15. Dispose of equipment and change bed linen if soiled.	Controls transmission of infection.
16. Measure client's body temperature.	Indicates response to therapy.
17. Record in nurses notes time that procedure was started and terminated, vital sign changes, and client's response.	Communicates care provided in an accurate and timely fashion.

Nurse Alert

If the client begins to shiver, discontinue the procedure. Shivering causes elevation in body temperature.

Client Teaching

Teach parents of small children how to perform a tepid bath in the home. Temperatures above 39° C or 102° F generally indicate the need for sponging. Adding alcohol to the water should be done only after instructions by the pediatrician. Adding alcohol to the water increases the risk of alcohol poisoning by inhalation.

Pediatric Considerations

A child's temperature can rise suddenly since his temperature regulation mechanisms are immature. Often the only warning sign is warm skin. It may be easier to immerse an infant or small child in a tub of tepid water than to actually sponge him. Exposure of all body parts simultaneously improves heat loss. Immersion also reduces the infants tendency to cry, which can increase body temperature. The child's head and shoulders should always be firmly supported during immersion.

Geriatric Considerations

The elderly client may have altered circulatory and heat conservation mechanisms. Peripheral vasoconstriction and muscular contraction (the shivering response) do not always occur normally following a drop in the environmental temperature. During sponging it is especially important to monitor an elderly client's body temperature since a decrease can occur quickly.

Female Perineal Care

Perineal care in women involves thorough cleaning of the external genitalia. The procedure can usually be performed during the bath. Most women prefer washing their perineal areas themselves if they are physically able. Perineal care prevents and controls the spread of infection, prevents skin breakdown, promotes comfort, and maintains cleanliness.

When a nurse provides perineal hygiene for the client, the nurse must wear gloves to reduce the risk of transmission of microorganisms, such as HIV or herpes from perineal drainage.

Potential Nursing Diagnoses

Potential for infection related to perineal secretions
Impaired skin integrity related to drainage or incontinence
Knowledge deficit regarding basic hygiene

Equipment

Washbasin	Bath blanket
Soap dish with soap	Waterproof pad or bedpan
Disposable or cloth washcloths (two or three)	Toilet tissue
	Disposable gloves
Bath towel	Disposable bag

Steps	Rationale
1. Explain procedure and its purpose to client.	Helps minimize anxiety during a procedure that is often embarrassing to both you and client.
2. Wash hands.	Reduces transmission of microorganisms.

Steps	Rationale
3. Pull curtain around client's bed or close room door. Assemble supplies at bedside.	Maintains client's privacy.
4. Raise bed to comfortable working position.	Facilitates good body body mechanics, which helps protect you from injury.
5. Lower side rail. Assist client to a dorsal recumbent position.	Provides easy access to genitalia.
6. Position waterproof pad under client's buttocks or place bedpan under client.	Prevents bedclothes from becoming wet.
7. Drape client by placing bath blanket with one corner between client's legs, one corner pointing toward each side of bed, and one corner at client's chest. Wrap bath blanket around client's far leg by bringing corner around leg and tucking it under hip. Drape near leg in same way. (Figs. 107, 108)	Prevents unnecessary exposure of body parts and maintains client's warmth and comfort during procedure.
8. Raise side rail. Fill washbasin with water that is approximately 41°-43° C warm (105°-109.4° F).	Rail maintains client's safety from accidental fall. Proper water temperature prevents burns to perineum.
9. Place washbasin and toilet tissue on overbed table. Place disposable or regular washcloths in washbasin.	

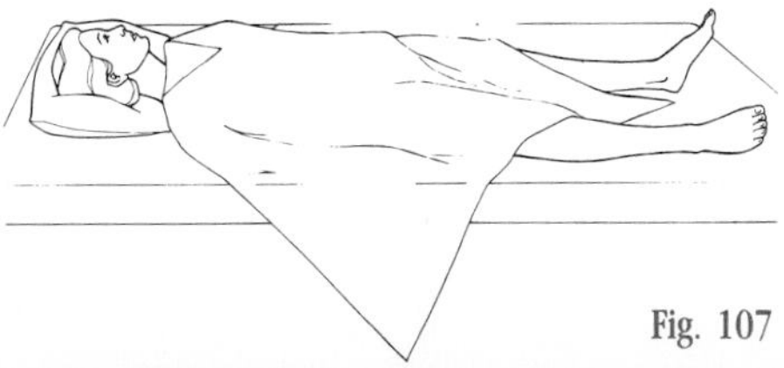

Fig. 107

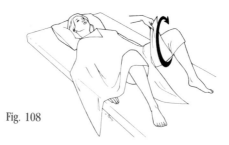

Fig. 108

Steps	Rationale
10. Lower side rail and help client flex her knees and spread her legs (a client with knee or hip disease may keep her legs straight).	Provides full exposure of genitalia.
11. Put on disposable gloves. Fold lower corner of bath blanket up between client's legs onto her abdomen.	Use of gloves minimizes transmission of microorganisms. Keeping client draped until procedure begins minimizes anxiety.
12. Wash and dry client's upper thighs.	Buildup of perineal secretions can soil surrounding skin surfaces.
13. Wash labia majora. Using your nondominant hand, retract labia from thigh. With dominant hand, wash carefully in skin folds.	Skinfolds may contain body secretions that harbor infection and cause body odor.
■ Wipe from perineum toward anus. Repeat on opposite side using different section of washcloth. Rinse and dry area thoroughly.	Reduces chance of transmitting microorganisms to urinary meatus.

Steps	Rationale
14. Separate labia with your nondominant hand. With other hand, wash downward from pubic area toward anus in one smooth stroke. Use different section of washcloth for each stroke. Pay particular attention to areas around labia minora, clitoris, and vaginal orifice. (Fig. 109)	Reduces chance of transmitting microorganisms to urinary meatus.

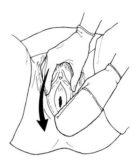

Fig. 109

15. If client is on a bedpan, pour warm water over her perineal area.	Rinsing removes soap and microorganisms more effectively than wiping.
16. Dry perineal area thoroughly.	Retained moisture harbors microorganisms.
17. Fold center corner of bath blanket back between client's legs over perineum. Help client off bedpan, lower her legs, and assist her to sidelying position.	Bath blanket prevents unnecessary exposure of body parts. Side-lying position provides easy visualization of anal area.
18. Clean anal area by wiping off any excess fecal material with toilet tissue. Wash area by wiping from vagina toward anus with one stroke. Discard washcloth. Repeat with clean cloth until skin is clear. (Fig. 110)	Cleaning prevents transmission of microorganisms.

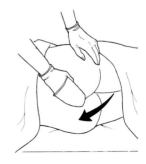

Fig. 110

Steps	Rationale
19. Rinse area well and dry with towel.	Retained moisture can cause maceration of skin.
20. Remove gloves and dispose of them in proper receptacle.	Moisture and body excretions on gloves can harbor microorganisms.
21. Assist client to comfortable position and cover her with sheet.	Making client comfortable minimizes emotional stress of procedure.
22. Remove blanket and dispose of all soiled bed linen. Return unused equipment to storage area.	Reduces spread of microorganisms.
23. Raise side rail and lower bed to proper height. Return client's room to its condition before procedure.	Side rail protects client from fall. Clean environment promotes client's comfort.
24. Wash your hands.	Reduces transmission of microorganisms.
25. Record in nurse's notes and report any observations (e.g., amount and character of discharge, condition of genitalia).	Timely recording ensures accurate documentation of care.

Nurse Alert

The presence of foul-smelling discharge may indicate an infection and require a physician's attention.

Clients with urinary or fecal incontinence, rectal or perineal surgery, or surgery involving the lower urinary tract, and women who are recovering from childbirth require special attention with perineal care. Care needs to be offered frequently.

Client Teaching

Adolescent girls should learn basic perineal hygiene and understand why they are predisposed to urinary tract infections.

Pediatric Considerations

A common problem among infants is diaper rash, created by the hot humid environment under the diaper. Airing and cooling are the most effective ways to promote healing. Change diapers as soon as they become wet. Remove excess clothing and occlusive diaper coverings.

Geriatric Considerations

Elderly women commonly have atrophy of the external genitalia along with a reduction in hair growth over the perineum.

Male Perineal Care

A male client requires special attention during perineal care, especially if he is uncircumcised. The foreskin causes secretions to accumulate easily around the crown of the penis near the urethral meatus. Penile cancer occurs more frequently in uncircumcised males and is believed to be related to cleanliness. Bacteria that collect under the foreskin act on desquamated cells to produce smegma, a substance irritating to the glans penis and prepuce.

As with the female client, the nurse should wear gloves when providing perineal care to the male. In addition, the male client requires perineal hygiene as a routine part of the bath, but also whenever urinary incontinence occurs and as a part of Foley catheter care.

Potential Nursing Diagnoses

Potential for infection related to urethral secretions
Knowledge deficit regarding basic hygiene care

Equipment

Washbasin
Soap dish with soap
Disposable or cloth washcloths
  (two or three)
Bath towel

Bath blanket
Waterproof pad or bedpan
Toilet tissue
Disposable gloves
Disposable bag

Steps	Rationale
1. Explain procedure and its purpose to client.	Helps minimize anxiety during a procedure that is often embarrassing to both you and client.

Steps	Rationale
2. Wash hands.	Reduces transmission of micro-organisms.
3. Pull curtain around client's bed or close room door. Assemble supplies at the bedside.	Maintains client privacy.
4. Raise bed to comfortable working position.	Facilitates good body mechanics and safety.
5. Lower side rail. Assist client to a supine position.	Provides easy access to genitalia.
6. Position waterproof pad under client's buttocks or place bedpan under client.	Prevents bedclothes from becoming wet.
7. Drape client by placing bath blanket with one corner between his legs, a corner pointing toward each side of body, and a corner over his chest.	Prevents unnecessary exposure before beginning procedure.
8. Raise side rail. Fill washbasin with water that is approximately 41°-43° C (105°-109.4° F).	Rail maintains client's safety. Proper water temperature prevents burns to perineum.
9. Place washbasin and toilet tissue on overbed table. Place disposable or regular washcloths in washbasin.	Equipment placed within your reach prevents accidental spills.
10. Lower side rail and don disposable gloves.	Reduces nurse's exposure to microorganisms.
11. Lower top corner of bath blanket below client's perineum. Gently raise penis and place bath towel underneath it.	Towel prevents moisture from collecting in inguinal area.
12. Gently grasp shaft of penis. If client is uncircumcised, retract foreskin.	Secretions capable of harboring microorganisms collect underneath foreskin.

Steps	Rationale
13. Wash the tip of penis at urethral meatus first. Using a circular motion, clean from meatus outward. Do not allow soap to get into meatus. Discard washcloth and repeat until penis is clean. Rinse and dry gently. (Fig. 111)	Cleaning moves from area of least contamination to most contaminated preventing entrance of microorganisms into urethra.

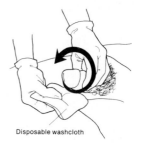

Fig. 111

Disposable washcloth

14. Return foreskin to its natural position.	Tightening of foreskin around shaft of penis can cause localized edema and discomfort.
15. Wash shaft of penis with gentle but firm downward strokes. Pay special attention to underlying surface of penis.	Vigorous massage of penis can lead to erection, which can cause embarassment for client.
16. Rinse and dry penis thoroughly. Instruct client to spread his legs apart slightly.	Spreading legs provides easy access to scrotal tissues.
17. Gently clean scrotum. Lift testicles carefully and wash underlying skinfolds. Rinse and dry.	Pressure on scrotal tissues can be very painful to client.
18. Fold bath blanket back over client's perineum and assist client in turning to a side-lying position.	Bath blanket maintains client's comfort and minimizes anxiety during procedure. Sidelying position provides access to anal area.

Steps	Rationale
19. Clean anal area by wiping off any excess fecal material with toilet tissue. Wash area by wiping from perineum toward anus with one stroke. Discard washcloth. Repeat with a clean cloth until skin is clear.	Prevents transmission of microorganisms.
20. Rinse area well and dry with towel.	Retained moisture can promote skin breakdown.
21. Remove gloves and dispose of them in proper receptable.	Moisture and body excretions on gloves can harbor microorganisms.
22. Assist client to a comfortable position and cover him with sheet.	Making client comfortable minimizes emotional stress of procedure.
23. Raise side rail and lower bed to proper height. Return client's room to its condition before procedure.	Side rail protects client from falling. Clean environment promotes client comfort.
24. Remove blanket and dispose of all soiled bed linen. Return unused equipment to storage area.	Reduces transfer of microorganisms.
25. Wash hands.	Reduces transmission of microorganisms.
26. Record procedure in nurse's notes and report any observations (e.g., amount and character of discharge, condition of genitalia.)	Timely recording ensures accurate documentation of care.

Nurse Alert

If a male client has an erection due to manipulation of the shaft of the penis, simply defer the procedure until later to avoid embarassing him. Thorough rinsing is necessary to remove soap, which can be very irritating to the urinary meatus.

Client Teaching

During perineal care the nurse can instruct the young male client on testicular self-examinations. Testicular cancer is the most common form of solid tumor in males between ages of 15 and 35.

Pediatric Considerations

In an infant the prepuce is normally tight for the first several months and should not be retracted for cleaning. Accidental tearing of the membranes may occur.

Geriatric Considerations

In elderly clients the testes diminish in size. This is a normal process of aging.

Nail and Foot Care

The nurse provides routine nail and foot care to prevent infection, foot odors, and injury to soft tissue. Often a client is unaware of a foot or toenail problem until pain or discomfort develops. The integrity of the feet and toenails is important to maintaining normal function of the feet so a person can stand and walk comfortably. The most common fingernail, foot, and toenail problems result from abuse or poor care such as biting nails or trimming them improperly, exposure to harsh chemicals, and wearing ill-fitting shoes. Disease, poor nutrition, and the physiological processes of aging also impair integrity of the nails.

Potential Nursing Diagnoses

Impaired skin integrity related to poor nail care
Pain related to poor nail care
Impaired mobility related to foot and/or nail disorders
Knowledge deficit regarding nail and foot care

Equipment

Washbasin	Emery board or nail file
Bath towel, face towel	Lotion
Washcloth	Disposable bath mats
Emesis basin	Paper towels
Nail clippers	Disposable gloves
Orange stick	

Steps	Rationale
1. Explain procedure to client.	Promotes clients participation in care procedures.

249

Steps	Rationale
2. Obtain physician's order if agency policy requires it.	During cutting, client's skin may accidentally be broken. Certain clients are more at risk of infection.
3. Wash hands.	Reduces transmission of micro-organisms.
4. Arrange equipment on overbed table. Pull curtain around bed or close room door.	Easy access to equipment prevents delays. Maintaining client's privacy reduces anxiety.
5. Assist client to bedside chair if possible. Place disposable bath mat on floor under client's feet. Place call light within client's reach.	Chair makes it easier for client to immerse feet in basin. Call light within reach assures his safety.
6. Fill washbasin with water at 43°-44° C (109°-110° F).	Warm water softens nails, reduces inflammation of skin, and promotes circulation.
7. Place basin on bath mat and help client place his feet in basin.	
8. Adjust overbed table to low position and place it over client's lap.	Easy access prevents accidental spills.
9. Fill emesis basin with water at 43°-44° C (109°-110° F) and place on paper towel on overbed table.	Warm water softens nails and thickened epidermal cells.
10. Instruct client to place his fingers in basin with his arms in a comfortable position.	Allows client to retain position.
11. Allow client's toenails and fingernails to soak for 10-20 minutes. Rewarm water in 10 minutes.	Softening of cuticles promotes easy removal of dead cells.

Steps	Rationale
12. Clean gently under finger-nails with orange stick. Remove emesis basin and dry fingers thoroughly.	Orange stick can be used to remove debris that harbors micro-organisms. Thorough drying impedes fungal growth and prevents maceration of tissues.
13. With nail clippers, clip fingernails straight across and even with tops of fingers. Shape nails with an emery board or nail file. (Fig. 112)	Cutting straight across prevents splitting of nail margins and formation of sharp nail spikes that can irritate lateral nail margins. Filing prevents cutting nail too close to nail bed.
14. Push the cuticle back gently with orange stick.	Reduces incidence of inflamed cuticles.
15. Move overbed table away from client.	
16. Put on disposable gloves and scrub callused areas of client's feet with wash-cloth.	Gloves prevent transmission of fungal infections to you. Friction removes dead skin layers.
17. Clean gently under client's toenails with orange stick. Remove feet from basin and dry them thoroughly.	Removal of debris and excess moisture reduces chances of infection.
18. Clean and trim toenails straight across. No not file corners of toenails.	Shaping corners of toenails may damage tissue.
19. Apply lotion to client's feet and then assist him back to bed and into a comfortable position.	Lotion lubricates dry skin by helping to retain moisture.

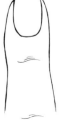

Fig. 112

Steps	Rationale
20. Make sure that call light is within reach. Raise side rail.	Call light and side rail provide for client safety.
21. Clean and return equipment and supplies to proper place. Dispose of soiled linen. Wash your hands.	Controls transmission of micro-organisms
22. Record procedure in nurse's notes and report any pertinent observations (e.g., breaks in skin or areas of inflammation).	Accurate documentation is timely and descriptive.

Nurse Alert

Clients with diabetes may have peripheral neuropathies causing reduced sensation. Therefore, test the water temperature carefully. Take extra care in trimming the nails of clients with diabetes mellitus or peripheral vascular disease. These clients tend to have poor wound healing capabilities and a slight cut could lead to serious infection.

Client Teaching

During nail care, instruct the client on proper techniques so routine care can be performed at home. Educate the client about safe use of home remedies for foot and nail care. Moleskin should be used to protect areas of the feet with corns or calluses. The moleskin does not cause local pressure as corn pads do. Chemical preparations used to remove corns can cause burns and ulcerations. Clients should be warned against cutting off corns or calluses since the risk of infection is great. Wrapping lamb's wool around toes can effectively reduce irritation to the skin.

Clients should also be taught about proper footwear. Socks can be worn to absorb perspiration. Footwear must always be clean to avoid infection. Women should be advised against wearing tight nylons or garters, which can constrict circulation. A person's shoes must not fit too tightly. It is recommended that a ¾-inch space between the great toe and the widest part of the shoe be present when a person stands. Clients should not try to cut hardened or hypertrophied nails. Referral to a podiatrist is a safer measure.

Pediatric Considerations

Infants and young children require routine trimming of fingernails and toenails to prevent cuts in the skin. Soaking is usually unnecessary. A child with short ragged fingernails may be a habitual nail biter. The presence of uncut nails with dirt accumulated under the edges is a sign of poor hygiene practices.

Geriatric Considerations

Elderly clients are more likely to have foot or toenail problems since poor vision, uncoordination, obesity, or inability to bend over can impede their performance of proper care. It is common for an elderly person to have dry feet and fissures of the feet and toes due to reduced sebaceous gland secretion and dehydration of tissue cells. The elderly also are more likely to suffer from conditions such as diabetes, heart or renal failure, and cerebrovascular accidents, all of which can contribute to foot and nail problems.

Care of Contact Lenses

Contact lens care is important to maintaining a client's optimal visual acuity and preventing corneal irritation or infection. Clients generally prefer to care for their own lenses when possible. However, illness may necessitate the nurse's assistance. Contact lens care includes cleaning, proper application and removal, and storage. Clients usually have a preferred method of caring for their lenses. When it becomes necessary for the nurse to assist with lens care, the client's preferences should be considered.

There are two major types of contact lenses: rigid and soft. Rigid lenses are thick and approximately 6 to 11 mm in diameter. Soft lenses are approximately 12.5 to 16.5 mm in diameter, large enough to cover the cornea completely. Soft lenses are flimsy because they consist primarily of water, 30% to 79% by weight (Carden, 1985). Both types are available as clear (untinted) or tinted lenses.

Potential Nursing Diagnoses

Pain related to corneal irritation

Altered visual perception related to decreased visual acuity

Knowledge deficit regarding contact lens care related to inexperience

Equipment

1. Prepare equipment and supplies for removal of lenses:
    a. Contact lens storage container
    b. Suction cup (optional)
    c. Sterile saline solution
    d. Bath towel
2. Prepare equipment and supplies for cleansing and insertion:

a. Lenses in storage container
b. Thermal disinfecting kit (optional)
c. Surfactant cleaner
d. Rinsing solution
e. Sterile lens disinfectant and/or enzyme solution
f. Sterile wetting solution for rigid lenses
g. Cotton ball or cotton-tipped applicator
h. Bath towel
i. Emesis basin
j. Glass of warm tap water

Steps	Rationale
1. Discuss procedure with client.	Client can assist in planning by explaining technique that may aid removal and insertion. Client may be anxious as nurse retracts eye-lids and manipulates lenses.
2. Have client assume supine or sitting position in bed or chair.	Provides easy access for nurse while retracting eyelids and manipulating lens.
3. Lens removal	

Removing Soft Lenses

a. Wash hands.	Reduces transmission of microorganisms.
b. Place towel just below client's face.	Catches lens if one should accidentally fall from eye.
c. Add a few drops of sterile saline to client's eye.	Lubricates eye to facilitate lens removal.
d. Tell client to look straight ahead.	Eases tipping of lens during removal.
e. Using middle finger, retract lower eyelid.	Exposes lower edge of lens.
f. With pad of index finger of same hand, slide lens off cornea onto white of eye.	Positions lens for easy grasping. Use of finger pad prevents injury to cornea and damage to lens.
g. Pull upper eyelid down gently with thumb of other hand and compress lens slightly between thumb and index finger.	Causes soft lens to double up. Air enters underneath lens to release suction.

Steps	Rationale
h. Gently pinch lens and lift out.	Protects lens from damage. Avoid lens edges from sticking together.
i. If lens edges stick together, place lens in palm and soak thoroughly with sterile saline. Gently roll lens with index finger in back and forth motion. If gentle rubbing doesn't separate edges, soak lens in sterile solution.	Assists in returning lens to normal shape.
j. Clean and rinse lens (see "Cleansing and disinfecting contact lenses"). Place lens in proper storage case compartment: *R* for right lens and *L* for left lens. Be sure lens is centered.	Ensures proper lens will be reinserted into correct eye. Proper storage prevents cracking or tearing.
k. Repeat Steps c-j for other lens. Secure cover over storage case.	Proper storage prevents damage to lens.
l. Dispose of towel and wash hands.	Reduces transmission of infection.

Removing Rigid Lenses

a. Wash hands.	Reduces transmission of microorganisms.
b. Place towel just below client's face.	Catches lens if one should accidentally fall from eye.
c. Be sure lens is positioned directly over cornea. If it is not, close the eyelids, place index and middle fingers of one hand behind the lens, gently but firmly massage lens back into place.	Correct position of lens allows easy removal from eye.

Steps	Rationale
d. Place index finger on outer corner of client's eye and draw skin gently back toward ear.	Maneuver tightens lids against eyeball.
e. Tell client to blink. Do not release pressure on lids until blink is completed.	Maneuver should cause lens to dislodge and pop out. Lid margins must clear top and bottom of lens until the blink.
f. If lens fails to pop out, gently retract eyelid beyond edges of lens. Press lower eyelid gently against lower edge of lens.	Pressure causes upper edge of lens to tip forward.
g. Allow both eyelids to close slightly and grasp lens as it rises from eye.	Maneuver causes lens to slide off easily.
h. Cup lens in your hand.	Protects lens from breakage.
i. Cleanse and rinse lens (see Cleansing and disinfecting contact lenses). Place lens in proper storage case compartment: *R* for right lens and *L* for left lens. Center lens in storage case, convex side down.	Both lenses may not have the same prescription. Proper storage prevents cracking, tearing, or chipping.
j. Repeat Steps c-j for other lens. Secure cover over storage case.	Proper storage prevents damage to lens.
k. Dispose of towel and wash hands.	Reduces spread of infection and keeps client's environment neat.

4. Cleansing and disinfecting lenses

Cleansing and Disinfecting Contact Lenses

a. Wash hands.	Reduces transmission of microorganisms.
b. Assemble supplies at bedside.	Provides easy access to supplies.
c. Place towel over work area.	Towel helps prevent lens breakage.

Steps	Rationale
d. Open lens container carefully, taking care not to flip lens caps open suddenly.	Prevents lenses from being accidentally spilled or flipped out of case.
e. After removal of lens from eye, apply 1-2 drops of daily surfactant cleaner on the lens in palm of your hand (use cleanser recommended by lens manufacturer or eye care practitioner).	Removes tear components, including mucous, lipids, and proteins that collect on lens.
f. Rub lens gently but thoroughly on both sides for 20-30 seconds. Use index finger (soft lenses) or little finger or cotton tip applicator soaked with cleaner (rigid lenses) to clean inside lens. Be careful not to contact or scratch lens with fingernail.	It is easier to manipulate and clean lenses using fingertips. Cleans all surfaces for microorganisms.
g. Holding lens over emesis basin, rinse thoroughly with manufacturer-recommended rinsing solution (soft lenses) or cold tap water (rigid lenses).	Removes debris and cleaning agent from lens surface.
h. Place lenses in storage case and fill with storage solution recommended by manufacturer or eye care practitioner.	Disinfects lenses, removes residue, enhances wettability of lenses, and prevents scratches from a dry case.

5. Lens Insertion

Inserting Rigid Lenses

a. Wash hands thoroughly with mild noncosmetic soap. Rinse well. Dry with clean lint-free towel or paper towel.	Lint or film on hands from soaps containing perfumes, deodorants, or complexion creams can be transferred to lenses and cause eye irritation.

Steps	Rationale
b. Place towel over client's chest.	Towel will catch dropped lens and avoid breakage, scratching, or tearing.
c. Remove right lens from storage case, attempt to lift lens straight up.	Sliding lens out of case can cause scratches on the surface.
d. Rinse with cold tap water.	Hot water causes lens to warp.
e. Wet lens on both sides using prescribed wetting solution.	Lubricates lens so that it slides easily over and adheres to cornea.
f. Place right lens concave side up on tip of index finger of dominant hand.	Proper manipulation of lens ensures easy insertion. Inner surface of lens should face up so that it is applied against cornea.
g. Instruct client to look straight ahead, while retracting both upper and lower eyelids; place lens gently over center of cornea. (Fig. 113)	Hard lens is rigid and can be placed as client looks straight ahead. Retraction of lids promotes easy insertion between lid margins.

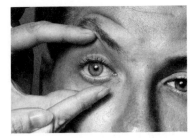

Fig. 113

h. Ask client to close eyes briefly and avoid blinking.	Helps to secure position of lens.
i. Be sure lens is centered properly by asking client if vision is blurred.	If lens slips to side of cornea or into conjunctival sac, vision will blur.
j. Repeat Steps c-g for left eye.	
k. Assist client to comfortable position.	Promotes client's comfort.

Steps	Rationale
1. Discard soiled supplies; discard solution in storage case; rinse case thoroughly and allow to air dry; wash hands.	Use of fresh solution daily prevents infection.

Inserting Soft Lenses

a. Wash hands with mild noncosmetic soap, rinse well, dry with clean lint-free or paper towel.	Lint or film left on hands from cosmetic or deodorant soaps can be transferred to lenses and irritate eye.
b. Place towel over client's chest.	Towel will catch dropped lens and avoid breakage, scratching, or tearing.
c. Remove right lens from storage case and rinse with recommended rinsing solution; inspect lens for foreign materials, tears, or other damage.	Removes disinfectant solution. Prevents irritation or damage to eye.
d. Check that lens is not inverted (inside out).	Soft lens is inverted if bowl has a lip; it is in proper position if curve is even from base to rim.
e. Using middle or index finger of opposite hand, retract upper lid until iris is exposed.	Soft lenses do not adhere as easily as hard lenses. Separating lids as much as possible allows room for lens to contact cornea without touching lids or lashes.
f. Use middle finger or the hand holding the lens to pull down lower lid.	
g. Tell client to look straight ahead and "through" the lens and finger, gently place lens directly on cornea, and release lens slowly, starting with lower lid.	Assures secure fit and comfort.
h. If lens is on sclera rather than cornea, tell client to slowly close eye and roll it towards the lens.	Maneuver centers soft lens over cornea.

Steps	Rationale
i. Tell client to blink a few times.	Ensures lens is centered, free of trapped air, and comfortable.
j. Be sure lens is centered properly by asking client if vision is blurred.	If lens slips to side of cornea or into conjunctival sac vision will blur.
k. If client's vision is blurred:	Technique repositions lens over center of cornea as client looks toward lens.
(1) Retract eyelids.	
(2) Locate position of lens.	
(3) Ask client to look in direction opposite of lens and with your index finger, apply pressure to lower eyelid margin and position lens over cornea.	
(4) Have client look slowly toward lens.	
l. Repeat Steps c-h for other eye.	
m. Assist client to comfortable position.	Promotes client's comfort.
n. Discard soiled supplies; discard solution in storage case; rinse case thoroughly and allow to air dry; wash hands.	Prevents infection.
6. Record or report any signs or symptoms of visual alterations noted during procedure.	May indicate presence of eye injury or disease. In most institutions it is not necessary to record procedure unless it was ordered or client is going to surgery.
7. Record on nursing care plan or Kardex times of lens insertion and removal if client is going to surgery or special procedure.	

Nurse Alert

A critically ill client admitted to hospital should be assessed for the presence of contact lenses. If they are present but not detected, they can cause serious corneal injury. Suction cups are available to lift a contact lens off the cornea.

Client Teaching

Clients who are relatively new wearers of contact lenses should be instructed in all aspects of lens care. Information to emphasize includes duration that lenses can safely remain inserted, cleaning methods, signs of corneal irritation, insertion techniques, and situations in which lenses should not be worn.

Pediatric Considerations

Parents or older children should learn all aspects of contact lens care.

Geriatric Considerations

Elderly clients who are able to wear contact lenses should be carefully assessed for their ability to insert and remove a lens. Any hand tremors or impairment in fine motor coordination or ability to grasp small objects may prevent them from performing self-care. If an older client suddenly becomes ill, a family member or friend should know how to remove contact lenses.

Care of Hearing Aids

A hearing aid intensifies the sound reaching the tympanic membrane (eardrum). Each client requires a different level of sound amplification. The aid consists of an ear mold, a battery compartment, a microphone and amplifier, and a connecting tube. The "behind-the-ear" device is the most common type used (Fig. 114).

Care of a hearing aid includes proper cleaning, battery care, and storage. The nurse must also know the correct way to insert a hearing aid for a dependent client.

Potential Nursing Diagnoses

Sensory alteration related to hearing impairment
Knowledge deficit regarding care of a hearing aid related to inexperience

Equipment

Emesis basin
Mild soap and water
Pipe cleaner (optional)
Syringe needle (optional)
Soft towel
Washcloth
Storage case

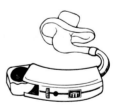

Fig. 114

Steps	Rationale
1. Wash hands.	Reduces transfer of microorganisms.
2. Assemble supplies at bedside table or sink area.	Prevents delays in procedure.

263

Steps	Rationale
3. Remove hearing aid from client's ear.	Eliminates unpleasant feedback squeal (harsh whistling sound), which can be caused by proximity of the aid to objects near wearer's body.
4. Determine if new battery is needed. ■ Close "battery door." ■ Turn volume slowly to high. ■ Cup hand over ear mold. ■ If no sound, replace battery and check again.	Batteries usually need replacing after 1 week of daily wear.
5. Check that plastic connecting tube is not twisted or cracked.	Cracked or twisted tube prevents transmission of sound.
6. Check to see if ear mold is cracked or has rough edges.	Can cause irritation to external ear canal.
7. Check for accumulation of cerumen around ear mold and plugging of bore (opening) in mold.	Prevents clear sound reception and transmission.

Cleaning

1. Detach ear mold from hearing aid.	Moisture entering battery and transmitter will cause permanent damage.
2. Add warm water and soap to emesis basin. Soak ear mold for few minutes. Be careful not to soak too long since cement holding ear mold to aid can become softened.	Removes cerumen that can accumulate on mold.
3. Wash client's ear canal with washcloth moistened in soap and water. Rinse and dry.	Removes cerumen and debris.

Steps	Rationale
4. If cerumen has built up in bore of ear mold, carefully clean hole with tip of syringe needle.	Wax will prevent normal sound transmission.
5. Rinse ear mold in clear water.	Soap may form residue that blocks opening in mold.
6. Allow mold to dry thoroughly after wiping with a soft towel.	Water droplets left in connecting tube could enter hearing aid and damage parts.
7. (Optional) Clean connecting tube carefully with pipe cleaner.	Removes moisture and debris, which can interfere with sound transmission and hearing aid function.
8. Reconnect ear mold to hearing aid.	Reassemble before inserting or storing hearing aid.

Storage

1. Open "battery door."	Ensures that there will be no contact, which would cause battery to run down.
2. Store hearing aid in storage case if client is about to do any of following: Bathe Walk in rain Use a hair dryer Sit in sun or under heat lamp Go to surgery or major diagnostic procedure Sleep Or is diaphoretic	Protects against damage and breakage.

Insertion

1. To reinsert hearing aid, first check battery and replace as needed.	Ensures proper sound amplification.

Steps	Rationale
2. Turn aid off and turn volume control down.	Protects client from sudden exposure to sound.
3. Place ear mold in external auditory meatus (ear canal). Be sure that ear bore in mold is first placed in ear canal. Shape of mold indicates which is correct ear. Slowly and with care, twist mold until it feels snug.	Proper fit ensures optimal sound transmission.
4. Gently bring connecting tube up and over ear toward back. Avoid kinking. Hearing aid fits around the upper ear.	Ensures correct function of hearing aid device and maintains client comfort.
5. Adjust volume gradually to comfortable level for talking to client in regular voice at a distance of 1-1.25 meters (3-4 feet).	Gradual adjustment prevents exposing client to harsh squeal or feedback. Client should hear you comfortably.
6. Remove soiled equipment from bedside and dispose of used supplies. Wash your hands.	Maintains clean environment and reduces risk of infection.
7. If client is going to surgery or other special procedure, record removal and storage in nurse's notes.	Protects you from liability if aid is lost.

Client Teaching

Discuss with the client guidelines for hearing aid use and tips for care: avoiding exposure to excess heat or cold, not dropping the aid on a hard surface, changing the battery over a towel or bed, not exposing the aid to moisture, not applying hair spray while wearing the aid, cleaning the battery to remove corrosion. The battery should be stored in a cool dry place. Keep the contacts clean by removing residue with a pencil eraser. Remove the battery when the aid is being stored.

Pediatric Considerations

A hearing deficit in children can cause serious developmental problems, including speech impediments, poor recognition of verbal cues, delayed socialization, and impaired learning.

Geriatric Considerations

Isolation and social withdrawal are common among persons with a hearing deficit. Often the elderly client is sensitive about admitting that he cannot hear clearly. The nurse should use good communication techniques to help the person understand what is being said.

Brushing and Flossing Teeth of Dependent Clients

Brushing, flossing, and irrigation are necessary for proper cleansing of the teeth. Brushing removes food particles, loosens plaque, and stimulates gums. Flossing removes tartar that collects at the gum line. Irrigation removes disloged food particles and excess toothpaste.

When the client is debilitated, the nurse must perform these skills for the client to ensure proper oral hygiene.

Potential Nursing Diagnoses

Altered oral mucous membranes related to poor oral hygiene
Pain related to gum irritation
Knowledge deficit regarding oral hygiene care

Equipment

Toothbrush with straight handle and small soft bristles
Toothpaste or dentifrice
Dental floss
Glass with cool water
Mouthwash (optional)
Straw
Emesis basin
Face towel and paper towels
Disposable gloves

Steps	Rationale
1. Wash hands.	Reduces transmission of micro-organisms.

Steps	Rationale
2. Place paper towels on over-bed table and arrange other equipment within easy reach.	Towels collect moisture and spills from emesis basin.
3. Pull curtain or close room door (optional if client only brushing teeth).	Provides client privacy. When brushing is part of bathing and total hygiene, privacy is essential.
4. Raise bed to comfortable working position. Raise head of bed (if allowed) and lower side rail. Move client or help client move toward you. Side-lying position can be used.	Raising bed and positioning client prevent nurse from acquiring muscle strain. Semi-Fowler's position helps prevent client from choking or aspirating.
5. Place towel over client's chest.	Prevents soiling of gown and bed linen.
6. Position overbed table within easy reach and adjust height as needed.	Easy accessibility of supplies ensures smooth, safe procedure.
7. Apply gloves.	Prevents contact with microorganisms in saliva.
8. Apply toothpaste to brush, holding brush over emesis basin. Pour small amount of water over toothpaste.	Moisture aids in distribution of toothpaste over tooth surfaces.
9. Hold toothbrush bristles at 45-degree angle to gum line. Be sure tips of bristles rest against and penetrate under gum line. Brush inner and outer surfaces of upper and lower teeth by brushing from gum to crown of each tooth. Use short vibrating strokes and brush each tooth separately. Clean biting surfaces of teeth by holding top of	Angle allows brush to reach all tooth surfaces and to clean under gum line where plaque and tartar accumulate. Back-and-forth motion dislodges food particles caught between teeth and along chewing surfaces.

Steps	Rationale

bristles parallel with teeth and brushing gently back and forth (Fig. 115). Brush sides of teeth by moving bristles back and forth.

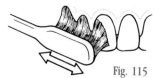

Fig. 115

10. Hold brush at 45-degree angle and lightly brush over surface and sides of tongue. Avoid initiating gag reflex.

Microorganisms collect and grow on tongue's surface. Gagging is uncomfortable and may cause aspiration of toothpaste.

11. Allow client to rinse mouth thoroughly by taking several sips of water, swishing across all tooth surfaces, and spitting into emesis basin.

Irrigation removes food particles.

12. Allow client to gargle or rinse mouth with mouthwash.

Mouthwash leaves pleasant taste in mouth.

13. Remove emesis basin and assist in wiping client's mouth.

Promotes sense of comfort.

14. Prepare for flossing by having client wash hands, if client is to floss independently.

Reduces transmission of microorganisms.

15. Prepare two pieces of dental floss approximately 25 cm (10 in) in length. Opinion differs over use of waxed vs unwaxed floss. Waxed floss frays less easily. Food particles adhere to unwaxed floss.

Need adequate length to grasp floss firmly and insert over surfaces of teeth.

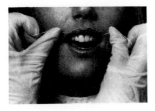

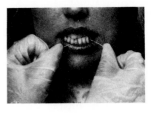

Fig. 116

Fig. 117

Steps	Rationale
16. Wrap ends of floss around the third finger of each hand. Using thumb and index finger, stretch floss and insert between two upper teeth (Fig. 116). Move floss up and down in see-saw motion between teeth from under gum lines up to top of each tooth's crown. Be sure to clean outer surface of back molar. Make a figure C around the edge of the tooth being flossed. Work systematically along each set of teeth.	Proper insertion and movement of floss along tooth surfaces mechanically removes plaque and tartar.
17. Take a clean piece of floss and wrap around third finger of each hand. Using index fingers stretch floss and insert between two lower teeth (Fig. 117).	Frayed floss becomes caught between teeth and can be torn off. This can lead to gum inflammation and infection. Position of hands helps reach lower tooth surfaces.
18. Move floss up and down, between gum lines and crown of lower teeth one at a time.	Upward motion of floss removes plaque and tartar.
19. Allow client to rinse mouth thoroughly with tepid water and spit into emesis basin. Assist in wiping client's mouth.	Irrigation removes plaque and tartar from oral cavity.

Steps	Rationale
20. Assist client to comfortable position, remove bedside table, raise side rail, and lower bed to original position.	Provides client comfort and safety.
21. Wipe off overbed table, discard soiled linen and paper towels in appropriate containers, remove soiled gloves, and return equipment to proper place.	Reduces transmission of microorganisms.
22. Wash hands.	
23. Record and report procedure in nurse's notes, mentioning specifically condition of oral cavity.	Documents response of client to hygiene measures.

Nurse Alert

All postoperative clients who receive general anesthesia are initially NPO after surgery and thus require frequent mouth care. Brushing is often contraindicated for these clients. Clients with sensitive gums or bleeding tendencies benefit from use of unflavored oral care sponges. A swab stick containing an aqueous solution of sorbital, sodium, carboxymethylcellulose, and electrolytes may be used.

Client Teaching

The client may be weak and unable to assist in his own care. However, the nurse can still provide instructions and answer any questions. She should discuss guidelines in the prevention of tooth decay: reducing intake of carbohydrates between meals, brushing within 30 minutes of eating sweets, always rinsing the mouth thoroughly with water, brushing and flossing before bedtime, and using fluoridated water if available.

Pediatric Considerations

A child's toothbrush should be approximately 21 cm (6 inches) in length.

Geriatric Considerations

Elderly persons can have reduced gum vascularity, decreased periodontal tissue elasticity, and brittle thin teeth. They also may have jaw bone atrophy. However, maintenance of regular dental hygiene should minimize periodontal disease.

Mouth Care for an Unconscious Client

The unconscious client poses special problems for the nurse with respect to mouth care. Many such clients have an absent or diminished gag reflex. Thus secretions tend to accumulate in the mouth, increasing the risk of aspiration. Critically ill clients often require an artificial airway and/or nasogastric tubes. These devices can cause considerable irritation to sensitive oral mucosal structures. Unconscious clients will require frequent mouth care to keep the mucosa well hydrated and intact.

Potential Nursing Diagnoses

Altered oral mucous membranes related to dried secretions
Potential for injury related to absence of gag reflex
Potential for infection related to gingival irritation

Equipment

Mouthwash or antiseptic solution
Toothettes or tongue blade wrapped in single layer of gauze
Padded tongue blade
Face towel
Emesis basin
Paper towels
Water glass with cool water
Petrolatum jelly
Suction catheter attached to suction

Steps	Rationale
1. Explain procedure to client.	Although unconscious, he may retain ability to hear explanation.

Steps	Rationale
2. Wash your hands and don gloves.	Reduces transmission of micro-organisms.
3. Place paper towels on over-bed table and arrange equipment.	Provides easy access to equipment.
4. Pull curtain around bed or close door to room.	Provides privacy.
5. Raise bed to its highest horizontal level. Lower side rail.	Use of good body mechanics prevents injury to both you and client.
6. Position client on side near you. Make sure that his head is turned toward mattress.	Protects client from aspirating secretions.
7. Place towel under client's face and emesis basin under his chin.	Prevents soiling of bed linen.
8. Carefully retract client's upper and lower teeth with tongue blade by inserting blade, quickly but gently, between the back molars. Insert when client is relaxed, if possible.	Prevents client from biting down on padded nurse's fingers. Provides access to oral cavity.
9. Clean client's mouth using toothettes or tongue blade moistened with mouthwash or water. Suction as needed during cleansing. Clean chewing and inner surfaces first. Swab roof of mouth and inside cheeks and lips. Swab tongue but avoid causing gag reflex if present. Moisten a clean applicator with water and swab mouth to rinse. Repeat as needed.	Swabbing stimulates gums and helps remove large food particles when brushing is impossible. Water or mouthwash provides lubricant for dry mucosa. Rinsing helps remove secretions and food particles. Suctioning minimizes risk of aspiration in clients with reduced gag reflex.
10. Apply petrolatum jelly to client's lips.	Prevents lips from drying and cracking.

Steps	Rationale
11. Explain to client that you have completed procedure.	Hearing and responsive capability are often still intact even in unconscious clients.
12. Remove gloves and dispose in proper receptacle.	Prevents transmission of microorganisms.
13. Reposition client comfortably, raise side rail, and return bed to its original position.	Maintains client's comfort and safety.
14. Clean equipment and return it to proper place. Dispose of soiled linen in "dirty" utility room.	Prevents spread of infection.
15. Wash your hands.	Reduces transmission of microorganisms.
16. Record and report procedure in nurse's notes, mentioning pertinent observations (e.g., presence of bleeding gums, dry mucosa, or crusts on tongue).	Accurate documentation should be timely and descriptive.

Nurse Alert

To ensure that any secretions in the client's pharynx are not aspirated, it may be helpful to have a second nurse assist with suctioning. Avoid the use of lemon glycerine swabs, which can cause drying of the mucosa and loss of tooth enamel.

Chemotherapy, radiation, and nasogastric tube intubation can cause stomatitis. Clients should rinse their mouths before and after each meal with a solution containing 0.5 to 1 teaspoon of salt to 1 pint of water (Wilson, 1986).

Geriatric Considerations

With aging there is reduced vascularity of the gums. In elderly persons the teeth may be brittle, drier, and darker in color. If dental hygiene is not maintained, inflammation and swelling of periodontal tissues can easily occur.

ELIMINATION

Female Urinary
Catheterization
Indwelling and Straight

Catheterization of the bladder involves the introduction of a rubber or plastic tube through the urethra into the bladder. The catheter provides for a continuous flow of urine in clients unable to control micturition or in those with obstruction to urinary outflow. Because in female clients the urethra is close to the anus, the risk of infection is always great and thorough cleaning of the perineum before catheter insertion is vital. Thereafter frequent perineal care must be provided.

Potential Nursing Diagnoses

Urinary retention related to perineal edema
Urinary retention related to infection

Equipment

Sterile catheterization tray
    Sterile gloves
    Sterile drapes, one fenestrated
    Lubricant
    Antiseptic cleansing solution
    Cotton balls or gauze sponges
    Forceps
    Straight or indwelling catheter
    Prefilled syringe with solution to inflate balloon for indwelling catheter
    Receptacle or basin (usually bottom of tray)
    Specimen container
Flashlight or gooseneck lamp
Sterile drainage tubing and collection bag

Tape, rubber band, and safety pin
Bath blanket
Waterproof pad
Trash bag
Basin with warm water and soap
Bath towel

Steps	Rationale
1. Explain procedure to the client.	Minimizes client's anxiety and promotes cooperation.
2. Raise bed to appropriate height.	Promotes use of proper body mechanics.
3. Close cubicle or room curtains.	Reduces client's embarrassment and aids in relaxation during procedure.
4. Stand on left side of bed if you are right-handed (or on the right if left-handed). Clear bedside table and arrange equipment.	Successful catheter insertion requires that you assume a comfortable position with all equipment easily accessible.
5. Raise side rail on opposite side of bed.	Promotes client's safety.
6. Place waterproof pad under client.	Prevents soiling of bed linen.
7. Assist client to a dorsal recumbent position (supine with knees flexed). Ask client to relax thighs so as to promote external rotation.	Provides good access to perineal structures.
8. Drape client with bath blanket. Place blanket diamond fashion over client: one corner over each foot, and last corner over perineum.	Unnecessary exposure of body parts is avoided, and client's comfort is maintained.
9. Wash perineal area with soap and water as needed, and dry.	Presence of microorganisms near urethral meatus is reduced.
10. Wash your hands.	Transmission of bacteria from your hands is prevented.

Steps	Rationale
11. If inserting indwelling catheter, open drainage system. Place drainage bag over edge of bottom bed frame. Bring drainage tube up between side rail and mattress.	Once catheter is inserted, you must immediately connect drainage system. Easy access prevents possible contamination. System is positioned to promote gravity drainage.
12. Position lamp to illuminate perineal area. (When using a flashlight, have another nurse hold it.)	Permits accurate identification and good visualization of urethral meatus.
13. Open catheterization kit according to directions, keeping bottom of container sterile.	Transmission of microorganisms from table or work area to sterile supplies is prevented.
14. Don sterile gloves.	Allows you to handle sterile supplies.
15. Pick up solid sterile drape by one corner and allow it to unfold. Be sure that it does not touch a contaminated surface.	Sterility of drape to be used as work surface is maintained.
16. Allow top edge of drape to form a cuff over both your hands. Place drape down on bed between client's thighs. Slip cuffed edge just under client's buttocks, taking care not to touch a contaminated surface with your gloves.	Outer surface of drape covering hands remains sterile. Sterile drape against sterile gloves is sterile.
17. Pick up fenestrated sterile drape and allow it to unfold as in Step 15. Apply drape over client's perineum, exposing labia and being careful not to touch a contaminated surface.	Fenestrated drape provides a clean work area near catheter insertion site.

Steps	Rationale
18. Place sterile trap and its contents on sterile drape between client's thighs.	Easy access to supplies during catheter insertion is provided.
19. Open packet containing antiseptic cleaning solution and pour contents over sterile cotton balls or gauze. (Be sure not to pour solution in receptacle that is to receive urine.)	All equipment is prepared before handling catheter to maintain aseptic technique during procedure.
20. Open urine specimen container, keeping top sterile.	Prepared to receive specimen.
21. Apply lubricant to bottom 2.5-5 cm (1-2 inches) of catheter tip.	Lubricant allows easy insertion of catheter tip through urethral meatus.
22. With your nondominant hand, carefully retract labia to fully expose urethral meatus. Maintain this position of your nondominant hand throughout remainder of procedure. (Fig. 118)	Full visualization of meatus is provided. Full retraction prevents contamination of meatus during cleansing. Closure of labia during cleansing requires that procedure be repeated.

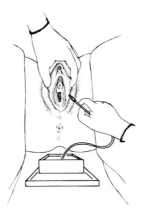

Fig. 118

Steps	Rationale
23. With your dominant hand, pick up a cotton ball with forceps and clean perineal area, wiping front to back from clitoris toward anus. Use a new clean cotton ball for each wipe: along near labial fold, directly over meatus, and along far labial fold.	Cleaning reduces number of microorganisms at urethral meatus. Using single cotton ball for each wipe prevents transfer of microorganisms. Preparation moves from area of least contamination to area of most contamination. Your dominant hand remains sterile.
24. With your dominant hand, pick up catheter approximately 7.5 to 10 cm (3 to 4 inches) from the tip. Place the end of catheter in the urine tray receptacle.	Collection of urine prevents soiling of client's bed linen and allows accurate measurement of urinary output. Holding catheter near tip allows easier manipulation during insertion into meatus.
25. Ask client to bear down gently as if to void and slowly insert catheter through meatus.	Relaxation of external sphincter aids in insertion of the catheter.
26. Advance catheter approximately 5-7.5 cm (2-3 inches) in adult, 2.5 cm (1 inch) in child, or until urine flows out catheter end. When urine appears, advance catheter another 5 cm (1 inch).	Female urethra is short. Appearance of urine indicates that catheter tip is in bladder or lower urethra. Further advancement of catheter ensures bladder placement.
27. Release labia and hold catheter securely with your nondominant hand.	Bladder or sphincter contraction may cause accidental expulsion of catheter.
28. Collect urine specimen as needed: ■ Fill specimen cup or jar to desired level (20-30 ml) by holding end of catheter in your nondominant hand over cup. With your dominant hand, pinch catheter to	

Steps	Rationale
stop urine flow temporarily. Release catheter to allow remaining urine in bladder to drain into collection tray. Cover specimen cup and set it aside for labeling.	
29. Allow bladder to empty fully (unless institutional policy restricts maximal volume of urine to drain with each catheterization).	Retained urine may serve as reservoir for growth of microorganisms. (Caution must be taken to avoid hypotension resulting from sudden release of pressure against pelvic floor blood vessels.)
30. With straight single-use catheter, withdraw it slowly but smoothly until removed.	Discomfort to client is minimized.
31. With indwelling catheter: ■ While holding with thumb and little finger of your nondominant hand at meatus, take end of catheter and place it between first two fingers of that hand.	Catheter should be anchored while syringe is manipulated.
■ With your free dominant hand, attach syringe to injection port at end of catheter.	Port connects to lumen leading to inflatable balloon.
■ Slowly inject total amount of solution. If client complains of sudden pain, aspirate back and advance catheter farther.	Balloon within bladder is inflated. If malpositioned in urethra, it will cause pain during inflation.
■ After inflating balloon fully, release catheter with your nondominant hand and pull gently to feel resistance.	Inflation of balloon anchors catheter tip in place above bladder outlet. (Fig. 119)

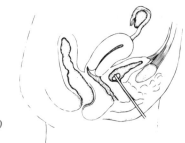

Fig. 119

Steps	Rationale
32. Attach end of catheter to collecting tube of the drainage system.	Closed system for urine drainage is established.
33. Tape catheter to client's inner thigh with a strip of nonallergenic tape. Allow for slack so movement of thigh does not create tension on catheter.	Anchoring of catheter minimizes trauma to urethra and meatus during client movement. Nonallergenic tape prevents skin breakdown.
34. Be sure that no obstructions or kinks are in tubing. Place excess coil of tubing on bed and fasten it to bottom bedsheet with a clip from drainage set or with rubber band and safety pin.	Patent tubing allows free drainage of urine by gravity and prevents backflow of urine into bladder.
35. Remove gloves and dispose of equipment, drapes, and urine in proper receptacles.	Transmission of microorganisms is prevented.
36. Assist client to a comfortable position. Wash and dry perineal area as needed.	Client comfort and security are maintained.

Steps	Rationale
37. Instruct client on ways to position herself in bed with catheter: side lying facing drainage system—catheter and tubing on bed unobstructed; supine—catheter and tubing draped over thigh; side lying facing away from system—catheter and tubing extending between legs.	Urine should drain freely without obstruction. Placing catheter under extremities can result in obstruction due to compression of the tubing from client's weight. When the client is on one side facing away from system, catheter should not be placed over his upper thigh; this forces urine to drain uphill.
38. Caution client against pulling on catheter.	
39. Wash your hands.	Reduces transfer of microorganisms.
40. Record results of procedure in nurse's notes, including size of catheter, character of urine, and client's tolerance.	Documents client's response and results of therapy.

Nurse Alert

If the catheter is mistakenly introduced into the client's vagina, leave it in place. Open a new sterile catheter and place it in the urethra (which is immediately anterior to the vagina). Then remove the misplaced catheter.

Women who are immediately postpartum, women who have had gynecological surgery, and clients who have just undergone bladder surgery are at risk for bladder distention.

Client Teaching

Instruct the client to keep the continuous drainage bag below the level of her bladder. This reduces the risk of urinary tract infections from backflow from the collection bag into the bladder. If the client is to be discharged with intermittent straight catheterization or with an indwelling (Foley) catheter, instruct her or a responsible person in catheter care, catheter insertion, and catheter removal.

Pediatric Considerations

Catheterization is most often used when urethral obstruction or anuria due to renal failure is believed to be the cause of the child's failure to void. Most female infants and children accommodate an 8- or 10-gauge French catheter. Special care must be exercised to restrain and reassure the child during the procedure.

Geriatric Considerations

Foley catheters should not be used in an older client who is incontinent. The nurse must modify the client's fluid intake patterns and must adjust toileting procedures to acommodate to a routine that will maintain proper fluid balance, independence in toileting, and integrity of the perineal skin.

Male Urinary
Catheterization
Indwelling and Straight

Catheterization of the bladder involves introduction of a rubber or plastic tube through the urethra and into the bladder. It is used for the following purposes: immediate relief of bladder distention, management of an incompetent bladder, obtaining a sterile urine specimen, and assessment of residual urine after voiding. Introduction of a catheter into a male client may be difficult if the prostate gland is enlarged. The nurse must not force a catheter through the urethra. Doing so might cause tissue injury.

Potential Nursing Diagnoses

Urinary retention related to enlarged prostate
Pain related to urinary retention

Equipment

Sterile catheterization tray
  Sterile gloves
  Sterile drapes, one fenestrated
  Lubricant
  Antiseptic cleaning solution
  Cotton ball or gauze sponges
  Forceps
  Straight or indwelling catheter
  Prefilled syringe with solution to inflate balloon for indwelling catheter
  Receptacle or basin (usually the bottom of tray)
  Specimen container
Sterile drainage tubing and collection bag

Tape, rubber band, and safety pin
Bath blanket
Waterproof pad
Trash bag
Basin with warm water and soap
Bath towel

Steps	Rationale
1. Explain procedure to the client.	Minimizes client anxiety and promotes cooperation.
2. Raise bed to appropriate height.	Promotes use of proper body mechanics.
3. Close cubicle or room curtains.	Reduces client embarrassment and aids in relaxation during procedure.
4. Stand on left side of bed if right-handed or on left side if left-handed. Clear bedside table and arrange equipment.	Successful catheter insertion requires that you assume a comfortable position with all equipment easily accessible.
5. Raise side rail on opposite side of bed.	Promotes client safety.
6. Assist client to a supine position with thighs slightly abducted.	Prevents tensing of abdominal and pelvic muscles.
7. Drape client's upper trunk with bath blanket and cover lower extremities with bedsheets, exposing only genitalia.	Unnecessary exposure of body parts is prevented, and client comfort is maintained.
8. Place bath towel under genitalia.	Prevents soiling of bed linen.
9. Wash perineum with soap and water as needed. In uncircumcised males, be sure to retract foreskin to clean urethral meatus. (Do *not* allow soap to get into meatus.)	Presence of microorganisms near urethral meatus is reduced.

Steps	Rationale
10. Wash your hands.	Prevents transmission of bacteria from your hands to meatus.
11. If inserting an indwelling catheter, open drainage system. Place drainage bag over edge of bottom bed frame. Bring drainage tube up between side rail and mattress.	Once catheter is inserted, drainage system is immediately connected. Easy access prevents possible contamination. System is positioned to promote gravity drainage.
12. Open catheterization kit according to directions, keeping bottom of container sterile.	Transmission of microorganisms from table or work area to sterile supplies is prevented.
13. Don sterile gloves.	Maintains asepsis throughout procedure.
14. Apply sterile drapes. Pick up solid sterile drape by corner and allow it to unfold. Be sure that drape does not touch a contaminated surface. Apply drape over client's thighs just below penis. Pick up fenestrated sterile drape, allow it to unfold, and drape it over penis with fenestrated slit resting over glans.	Sterility of drape as work surface is maintained.
15. Place sterile tray and its contents on drape alongside client's thigh or on top of thighs.	Easy access to supplies during catheter insertion is provided.
16. Obtain cotton balls or gauze with antiseptic solution. Open urine specimen container, keeping top sterile.	Prepares container for specimen.
17. Apply lubricant to bottom 12.5-17.5 cm (5-7 inches) of catheter tip.	Lubricant allows easy insertion of catheter tip through urethral meatus.

Steps	Rationale
18. With your nondominant hand, retract foreskin of uncircumcised male. Grasp penis at shaft just below glans. Retract urethral meatus between thumb and forefinger. Maintain nondominant hand in this position throughout procedure.	Firm grasp minimizes chance that erection will occur (if an erection develops, discontinue procedure). Accidental release of foreskin or dropping of penis during cleaning requires process to be repeated.
19. With dominant hand, pick up a cotton ball with forceps and clean penis. Move it in a circular motion from meatus down to base of glans. Repeat cleaning two more times using a clean cotton ball each time.	Reduces number of microorganisms at meatus and moves from least contaminated to most contaminated area. Dominant hand remains sterile.
20. Pick up catheter with gloved dominant hand approximately 7.5-10 cm (3 to 4 inches) from catheter tip. Hold end of the catheter loosely coiled in the palm of your dominant hand (optional: grasp catheter with forceps).	Holding catheter near tip allows easier manipulation during insertion into meatus and prevents distal end from striking a contaminated surface.
21. Lift penis to a position perpendicular to client's body and apply light traction. (Fig. 120)	Straightens urethral canal to ease catheter insertion.

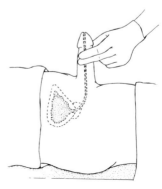

Fig. 120

Steps	Rationale
22. Ask client to bear down as if to void and slowly insert catheter through meatus.	Relaxation of external sphincter aids in insertion of catheter.
23. Advance catheter 17.5-22 cm (7-9 inches) in an adult and 5-7.5 cm (2-3 inches) in a young child, or until urine flows out catheter end. If resistance is felt, withdraw catheter; do not force it through urethra. When urine appears, advance catheter another 2 cm (1 inch).	Adult male urethra is long. Appearance of urine indicates catheter tip is in bladder or urethra. Resistance to catheter passage may be caused by urethral strictures or enlarged prostate. Further advancement of catheter ensures proper placement.
24. Lower penis and hold catheter securely in nondominant hand. Place end of catheter in urine tray receptacle.	Catheter may be accidentally expelled by bladder or urethral contraction. Collection of urine prevents soiling and provides output measurement.
25. Collect urine specimen according to Step 26 in female catheterization procedure (Skill 8-1).	
26. Allow bladder to empty fully (unless institutional policy restricts maximal volume of urine to drain with each catheterization).	Retained urine serves as reservoir for growth of microorganisms. (Precaution may prevent hypotension resulting from sudden release of pressure against pelvic floor blood vessels under bladder.)
27. With straight single-use catheters, withdraw slowly but smoothly until removed. Replace foreskin over glans.	Minimizes discomfort during removal. Tightening of foreskin around shaft of penis can cause localized edema and discomfort.
28. With indwelling catheters, inflate balloon and check for proper anchoring as in Step 31 of Skill 8-1.	Ensures that tip will remain in place above bladder outlet. (Fig. 121)

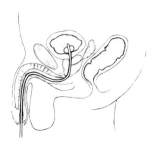

Fig. 121

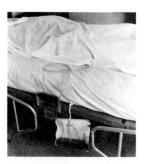

Fig. 122

Steps	Rationale
29. Attach end of catheter to collecting tube of drainage system.	Establishes closed system for urine drainage.
30. Tape catheter to client's inner thigh or lower abdomen (with penis directed toward client's chest). Use strip of nonallergenic tape. Provide slack so movement does not create tension on catheter.	Anchoring of catheter minimizes trauma to urethra and meatus. Taping to abdomen minimizes irritation at angle of penis and scrotum. Nonallergenic tape prevents skin breakdown.
31. Be sure that there are no obstructions or kinks in tubing. Place excess coil of tubing on bed and fasten it to bottom bedsheet with a clip to drainage set or with a rubber band and safety pin. (Fig. 122)	Patent tubing allows free drainage of urine by gravity and prevents backflow of urine into bladder.
32. Remove gloves and dispose of all equipment.	Prevents transmission of microorganisms.
33. Assist client to a comfortable position and wash and dry perineal areas as needed.	Promotes client comfort.

Steps	Rationale
34. Instruct client on proper positioning and the importance of not pulling on catheter (see Steps 32 and 34 of Skill 8-1).	Ensures unobstructed drainage through a closed system.
35. Wash your hands.	Reduces transmission of micro-organisms.
36. Record in nurse's notes results of procedure, including size of catheter, amount of urine drained, character of urine, and client's tolerance.	Documents client's response and results of therapy.

Nurse Alert

Do not force the catheter if resistance is met. In older men, prostatic hypertrophy may partially obstruct the urethra and prevent easy passage of the catheter. If resistance is met, notify the client's physician.

Client Teaching

Instruct the client to keep the continuous drainage bag below the level of his bladder. This reduces the risk of urinary tract infections due to backflow from the collection bag into the bladder. If the client is to be discharged with intermittent straight catheterization or with an indwelling Foley catheter, instruct him or his family on catheter care, insertion, and removal.

Pediatric Considerations

Male infants may not be able to accommodate the 8- or 10-gauge French catheters. In such instances a smaller soft plastic feeding tube may be used. Caution is necessary in catheterizing young males to avoid trauma that might result in sterility from damage to the ductal and glandular openings into the urethra.

Geriatric Considerations

Foley catheters should be avoided whenever possible in older adult clients who are incontinent. The nurse must modify the client's fluid intake patterns and schedule toileting procedures so a routine for bladder elimination will be developed that maintains proper fluid balance, independence in toileting, and skin integrity.

Applying a Condom Catheter

A condom catheter is an external urinary drainage device that is convenient to use and safe for draining urine in male clients. It is a soft pliable rubber sheath that slips over the penis, and it is suitable for incontinent or comatose clients who still have complete and spontaneous bladder emptying. The catheter may be preferred over an indwelling (Foley) type because drainage is maintained with less risk of infection.

Potential Nursing Diagnoses

Total incontinence related to impaired bladder function

Total incontinence related to decreased perception of sensation to void

Potential or actual impaired skin integrity related to exposure to urine

Equipment

Rubber condom sheath
Strip of elastic or Velcro adhesive
Urinary collection bag with drainage tubing
Basin with warm water and soap
Towel and washcloth
Bath blanket
Disposable gloves

Steps	Rationale
1. Wash hands.	Reduces transmission of micro-organisms.
2. Close door or bedside curtain.	Provides privacy.
3. Explain procedure to client.	Reduces client anxiety and improves cooperation.

Steps	Rationale
4. Don disposable gloves.	Reduces transmission of micro-organisms.
5. Assist client to a supine position. Place bath blanket over his upper trunk and cover his lower extremities with bedsheets so only the genitalia are exposed.	Supine position promotes comfort, and draping prevents unnecessary exposure of body parts.
6. Clean the genitalia with soap and water. Dry thoroughly.	Secretions that may irritate client's skin are removed. Rubber sheath rolls onto dry skin more easily.
7. Prepare urinary drainage bag by attaching it to bed frame. Bring drainage tubing up through side rails onto bed.	Easy access to equipment during connection of condom catheter is provided.
8. Grasp client's penis firmly along shaft with your non-dominant hand. With your dominant hand, hold condom sheath at tip of penis and smoothly roll sheath up onto penile shaft.	Firm grasp reduces chances that erection will occur. Condom should fit smoothly to prevent sites of constriction.
9. Be sure that tip of penis is 2.5-5 cm (1-2 inches) above end of condom catheter.	Allows free passage of urine into collecting tubing during voiding.
10. Encircle penile shaft with strip of Velcro or elastic adhesive. Be sure that strip touches only condom sheath. Apply snugly but not tightly. (Fig. 123)	Adhesive strip anchors condom in place. Snug fit prevents constriction of blood flow.
11. Connect drainage tubing to end of condom catheter.	Prevents soiling of bed linen and provides for collection of all voided urine.
12. Place excess coil of tubing on bed and secure to bottom bedsheet.	Patent tubing promotes free drainage of urine.

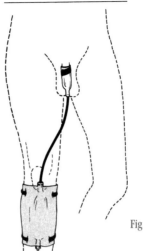

Fig. 123

Steps	Rationale
13. Dispose of soiled equipment and wash your hands.	Reduces transmission of microorganisms.
14. Record when condom catheter was applied and presence of urine in drainage bag.	Documents procedure. Also notes that client is able to empty his bladder and that urine is contained in drainage bag.

Nurse Alert

Adhesive tape should never be used to secure a condom catheter. It can cause constriction and reduction of blood flow to the penis. Velcro or elastic adhesive expands with changes in size of the penis and does not reduce blood flow.

Client Teaching

Occasionally the client will return home and wear a condom catheter intermittently or throughout the day. Instruct him and his family in perineal care, catheter application, and use of the optional leg bag.

Pediatric Considerations

Pediatric urinary collection bags are applied to the male infant or child when exact urinary output is required. The adolescent male may be catheterized only if there is no other method of obtaining exact urinary output.

Geriatric Considerations

Older men may require more frequent bladder emptying and should be offered the urinal or taken to the bathroom more frequently rather than subjected to condom catheter application.

Continuous Ambulatory Peritoneal Dialysis

Peritoneal dialysis is a type of dialysis in which the peritoneal membrane is used to promote the removal of fluid, electrolytes, and toxins from the client's blood. A form of peritoneal dialysis is continuous ambulatory peritoneal dialysis (CAPD). CAPD is a type of therapy that has made home dialysis feasible for the client with end-stage renal disease (ESRD). During this type of dialysis a permanent peritoneal catheter is surgically implanted into the peritoneal cavity and the principles of osmosis and diffusion remove fluid, excess electrolytes, and toxins from the client's blood (Perras et al, 1983). CAPD has the same three phases as routine peritoneal dialysis except the time cycle changes. The dwell time ranges from 4 to 8 hours. During this time an empty plastic bag and drainage tubing are folded and concealed under the client's clothes. After the dwell time the client drains the abdominal cavity, which is followed by a period of reinstilling fresh dialysate into the peritoneal cavity. CAPD requires changes in the dialysate ranging from three to five times a day. One major advantage of CAPD is that it allows clients to be out of the hospital, maintain their systems at home, and continue with daily activities. This method is not appropriate for all clients with ESRD and requires thorough education from nursing and routine follow-up in an outpatient renal clinic (Perras et al, 1983; Lane et al, 1982).

Potential Nursing Diagnoses

Fluid volume excess
Potential for infection related to peritoneal catheter

Equipment

Collect the following equipment for PD catheter site care:

- Sterile gloves   Maintains sterile asepsis.
- Occlusive dressing materials   Prevents entry of bacteria into
                                    PD site after treatment.

■ Hydrogen peroxide	Cleanse area around catheter site.
■ Providone solution	Anti-infective solutions and ointments reduce the risk for bacterial growth.
■ Providone ointment	
■ Mask	Reduces transmission of microorganisms.
IV pole	Placement of dialysate solution during the instilling cycle.
Y-connector tubing (CAPD clients may not need this tubing)	Allows the nurse to hang two warmed bags.
Sterile drainage bag	Permits proper collection of fluid from the peritoneal cavity during the drain cycle.

Steps	Rationale
1. Obtain client's weight.	Provides baseline information about weight attributed to fluid retention. A daily weight gain of 1 kg is equivalent to 1 liter of fluid.
2. Obtain vital signs.	Fluid volume changes associated with peritoneal dialysis increase the client's risk for hemodynamic blood pressure changes. This is especially true for clients having inhospital peritoneal dialysis.
3. Measure abdominal girth. ■ Mark midpoint of the client's abdomen. Maintain this mark as a reference for future abdominal girth measurements.	Provides baseline data regarding the amount of fluid in the client's peritoneal cavity.
4. Inspect catheter site for: Erythema Tenderness Drainage	Indicates possible infection at catheter entry site. Increases client's risk for peritonitis (Breckenridge et al, 1982).

Steps	Rationale
5. Measure client's body temperature.	Provides baseline data regarding client's febrile status.
6. Review hospital or dialysis unit's procedure for PD or CAPD.	There may be institutional variations regarding ordering of supplies; fill, dwell, and drain times; catheter care; discharge teaching plan.
7. Review physician's orders.	PD and CAPD require specific orders that are individualized to the client's fluid needs and disease process.
■ CAPD orders usually include three to five exchanges with a specific dialysate volume and composition as well as specific dwell time, which can range from 4 to 8 hours.	
8. Obtain laboratory data as ordered.	Documents client's fluid and electrolyte status and changes that occur from CAPD.
■ CAPD orders can vary, depending on individual client needs.	
9. Ordered dialysate at room temperature.	Dialysate that is too cold results in intolerance, cramps, or hypothermia.
■ Dialysate is warmed by placing solution bag on a warming pad, not into a warming solution.	Plastic dialysate bags are permeable. Immersing them in warm water when the protective wrapper is removed risks the introduction of bacteria from the nonsterile water. In addition, the osmotic concentration of the dialysate can change (Stangio, 1988).
10. Have a Deane prosthesis or PD button at the bedside.	Button is aseptically applied to the PD site at the end of the treatment. The button maintains patency of the insertion site for another treatment.

Steps	Rationale
11. Explain procedure to the client.	Assists in reducing anxiety and promoting cooperation.

Initiating the Dialysis Exchanges

Steps	Rationale
1. Wash hands.	Reduces transmission of micro-organisms.
2. Place client in semi- or high Fowler's position.	Instilling fluid into the peritoneal cavity decreases diaphragmatic excursion. These positions promote optimal lung expansion.
3. Make sure all clamps on the inflow and outflow tubings are in the "off" positions.	Prevents accidental instillation of air or dialysate into client's peritoneal cavity. Also prevents unscheduled removal of dialysate from the cavity prior to completion of ordered dwell time.
4. Add any medications as listed in the physician's order.	Medications can include: ■ Heparin to reduce accumulation of fibrin around the catheter tip. ■ Local anesthetic to dialysate aids in reducing back or abdominal pain related only to the infusion of the dialysate and no other causes (Birdsall, 1988). ■ Prophylactic antibiotics may also be ordered to reduce the risk of peritonitis.

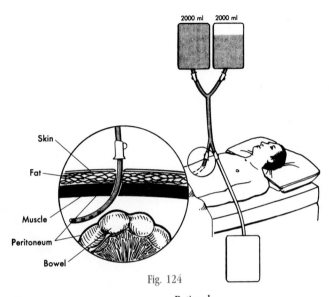

Fig. 124

Steps	Rationale
5. Attach two warmed dialysate bags to inflow tubing and attach to IV pole. (Fig. 124). Note that these bags are punctured exactly as IV solution bags (Unit 13).	Attachment of two dialysate bags promotes timely, organized follow-up exchanges. Standard peritoneal dialysis usually includes 24 exchanges. CAPD clients are instructed to hang only one bag because these clients have three to seven exchanges daily.
6. Prime inflow tubing by removing protective cap and maintaining sterility of the cap. Hold tubing over basin or sink, open inflow clamp, and allow fluid to run through the tubing until all air has been removed.	Maintaining sterility of the cap allows safe, sterile reapplication of cap on inflow tubing.\n\nPrevents air from entering the peritoneal cavity.
7. Open the clamp on dialysate bag. Infuse solution over prescribed time. Time usually includes 2 liters over 15 minutes.	Permits instillation of dialysate into the peritoneal cavity.

Steps	Rationale
8. Clamp inflow tubing for prescribed dwell time. ■ CAPD dwell time ranges from 3 to 5 hours. The CAPD client folds the tubing and infusion bag on the abdomen, which is concealed by clothing. The CAPD client uses the same bag and tubing for the drain cycle.	Clamping prevents air from entering the peritoneal cavity. This dwell time permits the peritoneal membrane to exchange fluid, electrolytes, and toxins from the client's blood.
9. Unclamp outflow tubing and drain; this usually is ordered for 20 minutes.	Permits drainage of dialysate and wastes from abdominal cavity. During the first two to three exchanges it is not uncommon for dialysate to remain in the cavity. However, this excess should drain with later exchanges.
10. Clamp outflow tubing.	Prevents untimed drain during subsequent exchange.
11. Empty and measure fluid in drainage bag.	Provides assessment of fluid balance of the dialysate solution. If a greater volume of fluid was infused than the amount drained, then the balance is a negative number. For example: 2000 ml of dialysate was infused and 1800 ml drained; then the balance is negative 200 ml (−200 ml).
12. When the exchange is complete either: ■ Cover catheter with a sterile cap. ■ Remove catheter and insert Deane button into catheter insertion site. This can be a medical procedure or designated to nurses in specialty units.	 Catheter remains in place if future PD is anticipated. Maintains patency of catheter insertion site.

Steps	Rationale
13. Inspect catheter dressing. If dressing is reapplied, use transparent occlusive dressing.	Dressing remains intact and dry, which reduces the risk of infection.
14. Wash hands and dispose of contaminated supplies according to agency policy.	Reduces transmission of microorganisms and blood-borne pathogens.
15. Document client's pre- and post-PD weight, abdominal girth, and dialysis fluid balance.	Notes the presence or absence of retained fluid in abdominal cavity.
■ Document client's vital signs before, during, and after dialysis.	Notes client's hemodynamic response.
■ Document temperature and status of catheter site.	Notes presence or absence of local or systemic infection.
■ Record color of drainage.	Notes any abnormalities in drainage color.
■ Record status of the catheter dressing or if new dressing was applied.	Provides a record of the status of the dressing's condition and most recent dressing change.

Nurse Alert

Stop dialysis and notify physician for change in vital signs, respiratory distress, bright red bleeding, fecal contents in the drainage, or scrotal swelling. These findings can indicate intolerance to the procedure, distention of the peritoneal cavity, perforation of the organ or vessel, perforation of bowel, or catheter displacement, respectively.

Complaints of cramps can indicate that the dialysate is too cold or being infused too rapidly. In addition, cramps can indicate the presence of an electrolyte imbalance.

Teaching Considerations

Clients who receive CAPD require meticulous teaching. These clients must be taught principles of surgical asepsis as well as the specific steps of their therapy. Prior to initiating CAPD a specific teaching plan is individualized for the client. The implementation of the teaching plan is usually done by specially prepared dialysis nurses and is based on national or regional teaching protocols.

Pediatric Considerations

Because small children are at risk for fluid and electrolyte imbalances, this therapy may not be selected. When it is used, it is selected for the adolescent in end-stage renal disease.

Geriatric Considerations

In the presence of other chronic diseases, the older adult may not be a candidate for this therapy. When it is selected, the nurse should do a detailed assessment of the client's learning needs and ability as well as the client's ability to implement the procedure in the home setting.

Continuous Bladder Irrigation

Continuous bladder irrigation is performed to maintain patency of the urethral catheter. This irrigation is maintained by way of a closed irrigating system (Fig. 125). The closed system ensures sterility of the irrigant and the irrigation system. Continuous bladder irrigation is commonly used in clients after genitourinary surgery. Such clients are at risk for small blood clots and mucous fragments that can occlude the urinary catheter.

Potential Nursing Diagnoses

Potential for infection related to indwelling catheter
Pain related to the presence of a catheter

Equipment

Sterile irrigating solution (as ordered by physician)
Irrigation tubing with clamp (with or without Y-connector)
IV pole
Antiseptic swab
Metric container

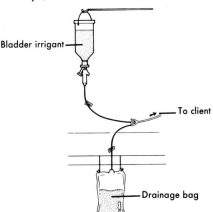

Fig. 125

Steps	Rationale
1. Explain procedure to client.	Reduces anxiety and promotes cooperation.
2. Close curtains or room door.	Provides privacy.
3. Wash hands.	Reduces transmission of micro-organisms.
4. Arrange client in a comfortable position, but one that does not occlude inflow or outflow tubing.	Maintains client comfort. Prevents accidental occlusion of drainage tubing and subsequent bladder distention.
5. Assess lower abdomen for signs of bladder distention.	Detects whether catheter or urinary drainage system is malfunctioning, blocking urinary drainage.
6. Using aseptic technique, insert tip of sterile irrigation tubing into bag containing irrigation solution.	Reduces transmission of micro-organisms.
7. Close clamp on tubing and hang bag of solution on IV pole.	Prevents loss of irrigating solution.
8. Open clamp and allow solution to flow through tubing, keeping end of tubing sterile; close clamp.	Removes air from tubing.
9. Wipe off irrigation port of triple-lumen catheter or attach sterile Y-connector to double-lumen catheter, then connect to irrigation tubing.	The third catheter lumen or Y-connector provides means for irrigating solution to enter bladder. System must remain sterile.
10. Be sure drainage bag and tubing are securely connected to drainage port of triple-Y-connector to double lumen catheter.	Ensures that urine and irrigating solution will drain from bladder.

Steps	Rationale
11. For intermittent flow, clamp tubing on drainage system, open clamp on irrigation tubing, and allow prescribed amount of fluid to enter bladder (100 ml is normal for adult); close irrigation tubing clamp, then open drainage tubing clamp.	Fluid instills through catheter into bladder, flushing system. Fluid drains out after irrigation is complete.
12. For continuous irrigation, calculate drip rate and adjust clamp on irrigation tubing accordingly; be sure clamp on drainage tubing is open and check volume of drainage in drainage bag.	Ensures continuous, even irrigation of catheter system. Prevents accumulation of solution in bladder, which may cause bladder distention and possible injury.
13. Dispose of contaminated supplies and wash hands.	Reduces spread of microorganisms.
14. Record amount of solution used as irrigant, amount returned as drainage, consistency of drainage in nurses' notes and I & O sheet. Report catheter occlusion, sudden bleeding, infection, or increased pain to physician.	Documents procedure and client's tolerance of it.

Nurse Alert

If the irrigant is too cold, bladder spasms can result, causing the client increased pain. If blood and blood clots are present, the nurse may need to seek an order to increase the rate of flow. The purpose of this intervention is to maintain catheter patency. Blood clots have the potential to occlude the catheter.

Teaching Considerations

Clients need to be instructed to observe the urine drainage for signs of blood or mucus, changes in color, or changes in consistency. In addition, clients are instructed to report increased frequency, duration, or intensity of bladder spasms and/or pain.

Geriatric Considerations

Continuous bladder irrigations are commonly ordered following prostate surgery. The majority of males needing this surgery are older adults. The older adult population has variable tolerances to analgesic agents, and the nurse must carefully assess the client's physiological and cognitive response to these medications.

Administering
an Enema

An enema is the instillation of a solution into the rectum and sigmoid colon. It is administered to promote defecation by stimulating peristalsis. Medications are occasionally given by enema to exert a local effect on the rectal mucosa. A cleansing enema can be used to soften feces that have become impacted or to empty the rectum and lower colon for diagnostic or surgical procedures.

Potential Nursing Diagnoses

Constipation, related to immobility or improper diet
Constipation related to medications slowing peristalsis
Self-care deficit: toileting, related to loss of voluntary muscle control

Equipment
Administration via rectal tube with container

Enema container
Ordered volume of solution warmed to 40.5°-43° C (105°-109° F) (with soap, salt, or other additives)
Rectal tube with rounded tip
Tubing to connect rectal tube to container
Regulating clamp on tubing
Bath thermometer to measure solution's temperature
Lubricating jelly
Waterproof pad
Bath blanket
Toilet paper
Bedpan or commode
Washcloth and towel
Disposable gloves

Administration via prepackaged disposable container

Prepackaged bottle with rectal tip
Disposable gloves
Lubricating jelly
Waterproof pad
Bath blanket
Toilet paper
Bedpan or commode
Washcloth and towel

Steps	Rationale
Rectal Tube with Container	
1. Explain procedure to client.	Reduces client anxiety and promotes cooperation during procedure.
2. Close room or cubicle curtains.	Provides client privacy.
3. Assist client into a left side-lying (Sims) position with right knee flexed. Children may also be placed in dorsal recumbent position. (Position clients with poor sphincter control on bedpan.)	Allows enema solution to flow downward by gravity along natural curve of sigmoid colon and rectum, thus improving retention of solution. (Clients with poor sphincter control will not be able to retain all enema solution.)
4. Place waterproof pad under client's hips and buttocks.	Prevents soiling of bed linen.
5. Drape client's trunk and lower extremities with bath blanket, leaving only anal area exposed.	Prevents unnecessary exposure of body parts and reduces client embarrassment.
6. Assemble enema container—connecting tubing, clamp, and rectal tube. Size of rectal tube should be 10-12 gauge French for infant or child and 22-26 gauge French for adult.	Rectal tubing should be small enough to fit diameter of client's anus but large enough to prevent leakage around tube.
7. Close regulating clamp.	Prevents initial loss of solution as it is added to container.

Steps	Rationale
8. Add warmed solution to container. Warm the water as it flows from faucet. Place saline container in basin of hot water before adding saline to enema container. Check temperature of solution with bath thermometer or by pouring small amount of solution over your inner wrist.	Hot water can burn intestinal mucosa. Cold water can cause abdominal cramping and is difficult to retain. *Maximum volumes for saline or tap water enemas (ml)* Infant 150-250 Toddler 250-350 School-age child 300-500 Adolescent 500-750 Adult 750-1000
9. Raise container, release clamp, and allow solution to flow enough to fill tubing.	Removes air from tubing.
10. Reclamp tubing.	Prevents further loss of solution.
11. Place bedpan near bedside unit.	To be easily accessible if client is unable to retain enema.
12. Wash your hands.	Reduces transmission of infection.
13. Don disposable gloves.	Prevents transmission of organisms from feces.
14. Lubricate 3-4 inches of tip of rectal tube with lubricating jelly.	Allows smooth insertion of tube without risk of irritation or trauma to rectal mucosa.
15. Gently separate buttocks and locate anus. Instruct client to relax by breathing out slowly through his mouth.	Breathing out promotes relaxation of external anal sphincter.
16. Insert tip of rectal tube slowly by pointing it in direction of client's umbilicus. Length of insertion varies: 7.5-10 cm (3-4 inches) for adult; 5-7.5 cm (2-3 inches) for child;	Careful insertion prevents trauma to rectal mucosa from accidental lodging of tube against wall. Insertion beyond proper limit can cause bowel perforation.

Steps	Rationale
2.5-3.25 cm (1-1½ inches) for infant. Withdraw tube immediately if it meets obstruction.	
17. Continue to hold tubing until end of fluid instillation.	Bowel contraction can cause expulsion of rectal tube.
18. Open regulating clamp and allow solution to enter slowly, with container at client's hip level.	Rapid infusion can stimulate evacuation prematurely before sufficient volume is infused.
19. Raise height of container slowly to appropriate level above anus (30-45 cm or 12-18 inches). Infusion time varies with volume of solution administered (e.g., 1 liter in 10 minutes).	Allows for continuous slow infusion. Raising container too high causes rapid infusion and possible painful distention of colon.
20. Lower the container or clamp tubing if client complains of cramping or if fluid escapes from anus around tube.	Temporary cessation of infusion prevents cramping. Cramping may prevent client from retaining all fluid.
21. Clamp tubing after all solution is infused.	Prevents entrance of air into rectum.
22. Place layers of toilet tissue around tube at anus and gently withdraw tube.	Provides for client's comfort and cleanliness.
23. Explain to client that feeling of distention is normal. Ask him to retain solution as long as possible while lying quietly in bed. (For an infant or young child, gently hold buttocks together for a few minutes.)	Solution distends bowel. Length of retention varies with type of enema and client's ability to contract anal sphincter. Longer retention promotes more effective stimulation of peristalsis and defecation. (Infants and young children have poor sphincter control.)

Steps	Rationale
24. Discard enema container and tubing in proper receptacle or rinse out thoroughly with warm water and soap if container is to be reused.	Controls transmission and growth of microorganisms.
25. Remove gloves by pulling them inside out and discard in proper receptacle.	Prevents microorganism transmission.
26. Assist client to bathroom or help position him on bedpan.	Normal squatting position promotes defecation.
27. Observe character of feces and solution (caution client against flushing toilet before inspection).	When enemas are ordered "until clear," it is essential to observe the contents of solution passed.
28. Assist client as needed to wash anal area with warm water and soap.	Fecal contents can irritate skin. Hygiene promotes client's comfort.
29. Wash your hands and record results of enema in nurse's notes.	Prompt recording improves documentation of treatment results.

Prepackaged Disposable Container

1. Follow Steps 1 through 5 for "Rectal tube with container."	
2. Place bedpan near bedside unit.	To be easily accessible if client unable to retain enema.
3. Wash your hands.	Reduces transmission of infection.
4. Don disposable gloves.	Prevents transmission of organisms from feces.
5. Remove plastic cap from rectal tip. Although tip is already lubricated, more jelly can be applied as needed.	Lubrication provides for smooth insertion of rectal tube without causing rectal irritation or trauma.

Steps	Rationale
6. Gently separate buttocks and locate anus. Instruct client to relax by breathing out slowly through his mouth.	Breathing out promotes relaxation of external anal sphincter.
7. Insert tip of bottle gently into rectum. Advance it 7.5-10 cm (3-4 inches) in adult. (Fig. 126) (Children and infants usually do not receive prepackaged hypertonic enemas.)	Gentle insertion prevents trauma to rectal mucosa.

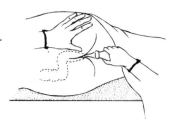

Fig. 126

8. Squeeze bottle until all solution has entered rectum and colon. (Most bottles contain approximately 250 ml.)	Hypertonic solutions require only small volumes to stimulate defecation.
9. Follow Steps 22 through 29 for "Rectal tube with container."	

Nurse Alert

If a client has an order for enemas "until clear," the nurse should not give more than three without verifying with the physician the need for more. Repeated enema administration can result in serious fluid and electrolyte imbalances.

Client Teaching

Clients should be instructed not to rely on enemas to maintain bowel regularity. Repeated use of enemas destroys defecation reflexes and leads to further alterations in bowel elimination.

Pediatric Considerations

The procedure for giving an enema to an infant or a child does not differ essentially from that for giving one to an adult. However, because of lack of motor control in the rectum, infants and small children may be unable to retain the instilled fluid. Plain tap water is rarely used in children because, being hypotonic, it can cause rapid fluid shifts and fluid overload. The Fleet enema is not advised for children because of the harsh action of its ingredients, which may produce severe diarrhea (leading to metabolic acidosis).

Geriatric Considerations

A frail elderly client may be more susceptible than a young adult client to fluid and electrolyte imbalances resulting from enema administration. Caution should be used when administering repeated cleansing enemas. In addition, the nurse should frequently monitor fluid and electrolyte status.

Removing Stool Digitally

Digital stool removal involves the introduction of the nurse's fingers into the client's rectum to break up a fecal mass and remove it in sections. This procedure is used when the fecal mass is too large to be passed voluntarily and enema administration is unsuccessful. Elderly or immobilized clients who are unable to ambulate regularly and who fail to maintain a balanced diet or fluid intake are susceptible to fecal impaction.

Potential Nursing Diagnoses

Constipation related to fecal impaction

Equipment

Water-soluble lubricant
Gloves
Bedpan
Waterproof pad
Bath blanket
Washcloth
Towel

Steps	Rationale
1. Measure client's pulse rate.	Serves as baseline for determining changes during procedure.
2. Explain procedure to client, noting that manipulation of the rectum can cause discomfort.	Explanation reduces client anxiety. Cooperation is necessary to minimize risk of injury.
3. Assist client to a sidelying position with knees flexed.	Provides access to rectum.

Steps	Rationale
4. Drape client's trunk and lower extremities with bath blanket.	Prevents unnecessary exposure of body parts.
5. Place waterproof pad under client's buttocks.	Prevents soiling of bed linen.
6. Place bedpan next to client.	To be receptacle for stool.
7. Don disposable gloves.	Prevents transmission of micro-organisms.
8. Lubricate your gloved index finger with ample amount of lubricating jelly.	Permits smooth insertion of finger into rectum.
9. Insert your finger into client's rectum and advance it slowly along rectal wall toward umbilicus.	Allows you to reach impacted stool high in rectum.
10. Gently loosen fecal mass by massaging around it. Work finger into hardened core.	Loosening mass allows you to penetrate it with less discomfort to client.
11. Work stool downward toward anus. Remove small sections of feces at a time.	Prevents need to force finger up into rectum and minimizes trauma to mucosa.
12. Periodically assess client's heart rate and look for signs of fatigue. Stop procedure if client's heart rate drops or rhythm changes.	Vagal stimulation slows heart rate. Procedure may exhaust client.
13. Continue to clear rectum of feces and allow client to rest at intervals.	Rest improves client's tolerance of procedure.
14. After disimpaction, use washcloth and towel to wash buttocks and anal area.	Promotes client's sense of comfort and cleanliness.
15. Remove bedpan and dispose of feces. Remove gloves by turning them inside out and discard in proper receptacle.	Prevents transmission of micro-organisms.

Steps	Rationale
16. Assist client to toilet or a clean bedpan.	Disimpaction may stimulate defecation reflex.
17. Wash your hands and record in nurse's notes results of disimpaction. Describe fecal characteristics. (Procedure may be followed by enemas or cathartics.)	Prompt recording improves accuracy of documentation.

Nurse Alert

Excessive rectal manipulation can cause irritation to the mucosa, bleeding, and stimulation of the vagus nerve. When there is vagal stimulation, a reflexive slowing of the heart rate occurs and can cause dangerous dysrhythmias in some clients.

Client Teaching

Clients and their families should be instructed how to avoid fecal impactions—by modifying their diets to include more fruits and vegetables, by increasing their fluid intake (if not contraindicated), and by altering sedentary activity patterns.

Pediatric Considerations

Digital removal of stool is rarely needed in children. If it does become necessary, it should be preceded by a careful explanation to both the parent and the child. Preventive measures are more common and include stool softeners, diet changes, and adequate hydration.

Geriatric Considerations

In the older adult population, constipation tends to be more a problem than in younger persons, and along with it the more frequent use of laxatives and/or enemas. In addition, there is a higher percentage of elderly clients with chronic cardiovascular disease, which puts these persons at greater risk of dysrhythmias induced by vagal stimulation during digital stool removal.

CARE OF THE SURGICAL CLIENT

Demonstrating
Postoperative Exercises

The manner in which the nurse prepares a client for surgery can have a positive influence on his recovery. With well-planned instruction a client can learn how to cough and deep breathe regularly, ambulate and resume activities of daily living early after surgery, and participate in the recovery process to attain a sense of well-being. A few simple maneuvers—diaphragmatic breathing, coughing, turning, and leg exercises—serve to prevent respiratory and circulatory complications that otherwise might develop in a client who stays inactive postoperatively. The exercises are important for any client undergoing general anesthesia.

Diaphragmatic breathing promotes lung expansion and helps clear respiratory passages of anesthetic gases. Coughing assists in removing retained mucus that accumulates in the airways because of depressed respirations and anesthesia. Leg exercises and turning improve blood flow to the lower extremities, thus reducing venous stasis.

When the nurse plans postoperative exercises, it is important to know the client's risks of complications. Chronic smoking, a history of respiratory disease, and a painful surgical incision all can contribute to impairing a client's ventilatory capacity. Likewise, a history of peripheral vascular disease or forced immobilization from an applied cast or traction can increase the risk of poor circulatory perfusion. By helping clients learn how to participate actively in postoperative recovery the nurse provides an effective and preventive plan of care.

Potential Nursing Diagnoses

Ineffective airway clearance related to incisional pain
Ineffective airway clearance related to reduced consciousness
Pain related to surgical incision
Impaired physical mobility related to pain

Impaired physical mobility related to imposed restrictions of movement

Equipment

Pillow (optional)

Steps	Rationale

Diaphragmatic Breathing

Demonstrate the following steps to client:

1. Sit or stand upright, placing your hands palm down along lower borders of your anterior rib cage. (Fig. 127)

Upright position facilitates diaphragmatic excursion. This placement of hands allows individual to feel movement of chest and abdomen as diaphragm descends and lungs expand.

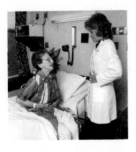

Fig. 127

2. Take slow deep breath, inhaling through your nose.

Discourages panting or hyperventilation. Breathing through nose warms, humidifies, and filters air.

3. Give attention to normal downward movement of your diaphragm during inspiration. Abdominal organs descend, and thorax expands slowly.

Your explanation focuses on normal ventilatory movements so the client can anticipate how diaphragmatic breathing feels.

4. Avoid using your chest and shoulders while inhaling.

Use of auxiliary chest and shoulder muscles increases energy expenditure during breathing.

Steps	Rationale
5. After holding your breath to a count of 3, slowly exhale through your mouth.	Allows gradual expulsion of all air.
6. Repeat exercise three to five times.	Establishes slow rhythmical breathing pattern.
7. Have client practice exercise.	Reinforces learning.

Coughing

Demonstrate the following steps to client:

1. Assume an upright position in bed or on side of bed.	Facilitates diaphragmatic movement and enhances expansion of lungs.
2. Take two or three slow diaphragmatic breaths.	Expands lungs fully to move air behind mucus in airways.
3. Inhale deeply, hold your breath to count of 3, and cough once and then again.	Two successive coughs help remove mucus more effectively and completely than one forceful cough.
4. Do not merely clear your throat.	Clearing of throat does not remove mucus from deep in airways.
5. If surgical incision is to be in chest or abdominal area, place one hand over the incisional area and other hand on top of first. During inhalation and coughing, press gently against that area to splint incision. (A pillow over incision is optional.) (Fig. 128)	Surgical incision results in cutting of muscles and tissues. Breathing and coughing place strain on a suture line and cause discomfort. Splinting minimizes incisional pulling. Hands provide firm support to incision.

Fig. 128

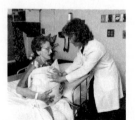

Steps	Rationale
6. Have client practice coughing with splinting.	You are trying to emphasize value of deep coughing with splinting to effectively expectorate mucus with minimal discomfort.

Turning

NOTE: This is for turning client to his left side.

1. Instruct client to assume a supine position on right half of bed. (Side rails should be up on both sides.)	You cannot demonstrate exercise in client's bed for obvious reasons of asepsis. Positioning begins toward right side of bed so turning to left will not cause client to roll toward bed's edge.
2. Place client's left hand over incisional area for splinting.	Supports incisional area to minimize pulling of suture line during turning.
3. Have client keep his left leg straight and flex right knee up and over left leg.	Straight left leg stabilizes client's position. Flexed right leg shifts weight for easier turning.
4. Grasping side rail on left side of bed with his right hand, client pulls toward left and rolls onto his left side.	Minimizes effort needed to turn.

Leg Exercises

NOTE: If client's surgery involves one or both extremities, a surgeon's order is required before exercises can be performed postoperatively. Legs unaffected by surgery can be safely exercised unless a client has preexisting alterations.

1. Place client supine in bed. Demonstrate leg exercises by putting him through passive range of motion.	Provides for normal anatomical position of lower extremities.

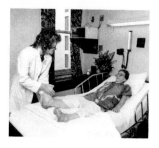

Fig. 129

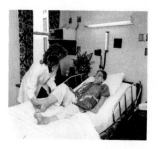

Fig. 130

Steps	Rationale
2. Instruct client to rotate each ankle in a complete circle by pretending to draw circles with his big toe. (Fig. 129)	Maintains joint mobility and promotes venous return.
3. Alternate dorsiflexion and plantar flexion of the feet. Client will feel his calf muscles first contract and then relax.	Stretches and contracts gastrocnemius muscles.
4. Have client flex and extend his knees. (Fig. 130)	
5. Keeping his legs straight, client then alternately raises each leg from surface of bed and lets it drop gently.	Promotes contraction and relaxation of quadriceps muscles.

Nurse Alert

Know whether a client will be allowed to do active exercising of his extremities postoperatively. Some vascular procedures, such as repair of the femoral-popliteal artery, prohibit active exercising until the vascular graft has healed. Likewise, certain procedures may contraindicate turning.

Client Teaching

The nurse must demonstrate each exercise carefully and then have the client practice doing it under supervision. Eventually the client should be able to perform the exercises independently. During a routine postoperative day it is hoped that he will become able to initiate exercises on his own.

Pediatric Considerations

Children usually are at lower risk of postoperative complications because they tend to resume activity quickly. However, seriously ill children may require guidance and support. Parents can be helpful in demonstrating and reinforcing exercises.

Geriatric Considerations

Elderly persons usually are at greater risk of postoperative complications because of the aging process. They often have increased calcium and cholesterol deposits in small arteries, and vessel walls thicken. These changes predispose to clot formation. The elderly person's rib cage also tends to stiffen and diaphragmatic movement declines, reducing lung expansion. It often takes longer for an elderly client to become oriented following surgery due to neurological and sensory changes. Thus active participation in exercises may be lessened.

Surgical Skin
Preparation

Before any surgical procedure, the skin is prepared so the number of resident microorganisms that could enter a surgical wound will be minimized. Skin preparation routinely requires thorough cleaning with scrubs and/or showers. Hair clipping or shaving may also be performed to remove body hair that harbors microorganisms and obstructs the view of the surgical field. An area of skin larger than the actual surgical site is always prepared to ensure that the surgical site is as clean as possible.

Although some physicians order a preoperative shave the night before surgery, it is preferable to shave hair immediately before surgery. Hair removal can injure the skin, especially if a razor is used. Minor nicks or cuts in the skin are prime sites for bacterial growth. The longer the period between the shave and surgery, the greater is the potential for bacterial growth.

Potential Nursing Diagnoses

Potential for infection related to skin cuts
Impaired skin integrity related to razor cuts
Pain related to skin abrasions or cuts

Equipment

Clipping
    Electric clippers
    Scissors
    Towel
    Cotton balls, applicators, and antiseptic solution (optional)
Wet Shave
    Razor with extra blade
    Clean basin with warm water
    Gauze sponges

Basin with liquid antiseptic soap mixed with water
Waterproof underpad or towels
Cotton balls, cotton applicators, and antiseptic solution (op-
tional)
Disposable gloves (optional)
Portable lamp
Bath blanket

Steps	Rationale
1. Inspect general condition of skin.	If lesions, irritations, or signs of skin infection are present, shaving should not be done. These conditions increase chances for postoperative wound infections.
2. Review physician's order for area to be clipped (Review institution's operating room manual as needed.)	Extent of area for hair removal depends upon site of incision, nature of surgery, and physician's preference. Area is always larger than actual incision to ensure wide perimeter with minimal bacteria.
3. Explain procedure and rationale for removal of hair over large surface area.	Promotes cooperation and minimizes anxiety because client may think incision will be as large as clipped site.
4. Wash hands.	Reduces transmission of infection.
5. Close room doors or bedside curtains.	Provides client privacy.
6. Raise bed to high position.	Avoids need to bend over for long periods of time.
7. Position client comfortably with surgical site accessible.	Hair removal and skin preparation can take several minutes. Nurse should have easy access to hard-to-reach areas.
8. Hair clipping: ■ Lightly dry area to be clipped with towel.	Removes moisture, which interferes with clean cut of clippers.

Steps	Rationale
■ Hold clippers in dominant hand, about 1 cm above skin, and cut hair in direction it grows. Clip small area at time.	Prevents pulling on hair and abrasion of skin.
■ Arrange drapes as necessary.	Prevents unnecessary exposure of body parts.
■ Lightly brush off cut hair with towel.	Removes contaminated hair and promotes client's comfort. Improves visibility of area being clipped.
■ When clipped area is over body crevices, (for example, umbilicus or groin), clean crevices with cotton-tipped applicators or cotton ball dipped in antiseptic solution, then dry.	Removes secretions, dirt, and any remaining hair clippings, which harbor microorganisms.

9. Wet shave

■ Place towel or waterproof pads under body part to be shaved.	Prevents soiling of bed linen.
■ Drape client with bath blanket, leaving only area to be shaved at one time (10-20 cm [4-8 in]) exposed.	Prevents unnecessary exposure of body parts and reduces client's anxiety.
■ Adjust lamp.	Provides maximum skin illumination.
■ Apply gloves if desired.	Prevents exposure to blood resulting from accidental cuts.
■ Lather skin with gauze sponges dipped in antiseptic soap.	Softens hair and reduces friction from razor.
■ Shave small area at a time. With nondominant hand hold gauze sponge to stabilize skin. Hold razor at 45-degree angle in dominant hand and	Shaving small areas minimizes cutting skin; shaving in direction hair grows prevents pulling.

Steps	Rationale

shave hair in direction it
grows. Use short, gentle
strokes. (Fig. 131)

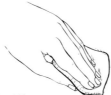

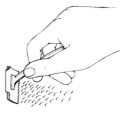

Fig. 131

- Rinse razor in basin of water as soap and hair accumulate on the blade. Change and discard blades as they become dull.

  Maintains clean, sharp razor edge to promote client's comfort.

- Rearrange bath blanket as each portion of shave is completed.

  Maintains client's comfort and privacy.

- Use washcloth and warm water to rinse away remaining hair and soap solution. Change water as needed.

  Reduces skin irritation and improves visibility of skin.

- If shaved area is over body crevices (for example, umbilicus or groin), cleanse with cotton tipped applicators or cotton balls dipped in antiseptic solution.

  Removes secretions, dirt, and other remaining hair clippings, which harbor microorganisms.

- Dry crevices with cotton balls or applicators.

  Reduces maceration of skin from retained moisture.

- Discard waterproof towel or pad.

  Reduces spread of microorganisms.

- Observe skin closely for nicks or cuts.

  Any break in skin integrity increases risk of wound infection.

10. Tell client that procedure is completed.

    Relieves client's anxiety.

Steps	Rationale
11. Clean and dispose of equipment according to policy and dispose of gloves.	Proper disposal of soiled equipment prevents spread of infection and reduces risk of injury from razor blades.
12. Inspect condition of skin after completion of hair removal.	Determines if there is remaining hair or if skin was cut.
13. Record procedure, area clipped or shaved, and condition of skin before and after in nurse's notes.	Documents procedure performed and condition of skin before surgery.

Nurse Alert

Use extra caution if the client has a preexisting bleeding tendency such as leukemia, aplastic anemia, or hemophilia or has been receiving anticoagulant therapy. If a client has a bleeding tendency or is on anticoagulant therapy, dry shaving may be ordered.

Client Teaching

Explain the purpose of shaving and its importance to the client's welfare. The client should understand that it is necessary to shave a larger surface area than the immediate surgical site. He may fear that the surgical incision will be as large as the shaved area.

Pediatric Considerations

A shave will sometimes be deferred because the amount of body hair on a young child is limited. An adolescent has more body hair and may need to undergo a shave.

Geriatric Considerations

The elderly client's skin can be thin and fragile. Use caution when shaving to avoid cuts.

NUTRITION

Insertion, Placement, and Anchoring of Nasogastic Tubes

Large-bore and small-bore

Insertion of a nasogastric tube involves placing a pliable plastic tube through the client's nasopharynx into the stomach. The tube has a hollow lumen that allows both the removal of gastric secretions from and the introduction of solutions into the stomach.

Potential Nursing Diagnoses

Pain related to NG tube placement

Altered nutrition less than body requirements related to reduced caloric intake

Impaired skin integrity related to pressure of NG tube at naris

Equipment

Large-bore tube placement
   NG tube (14-18 French)
   Water-soluble lubricant
   60 ml catheter tip syringe
   Stethoscope
   Hypoallergenic tape and tincture of benzoin
   Glass of water and straw
   Emesis basin
   Tongue blade
   Towel
   Clean gloves
   Facial tissue
   Normal saline solution

Small-bore tube placement
  NG tube (8-12 French)
  30 ml or larger luer-lok or tip syringe
  Stethoscope
  Hypoallergenic tape and tincture of benzoin
  Glass of water and straw
  Emesis basin
  Tongue blade
  Towel
  Guidewire or stylet
  Facial tissues
  Clean gloves
  pH tape

Steps	Rationale
Tube Insertion	
1. Explain the procedure fully to client, as well as purpose of nasogastric decompression.	Procedure is easier to complete with client's full cooperation.
2. Wash hands.	Reduces transfer of microorganisms.
3. Assemble all equipment at bedside.	Organized procedure can be performed in a timely fashion, limiting client's discomfort.
4. Assist client to high Fowler position with pillows behind head and shoulders.	Promotes client's ability to swallow.
5. Place bath towel over client's chest. Keep facial tissues within client's reach.	Prevents soiling of client's gown. Insertion of tube through nasal passages may cause tearing.
6. Stand on right side of bed if you are right handed (or on left side if left-handed).	Allows easier manipulating of tubing.
7. Instruct client to relax and breathe normally while occluding one naris. Then repeat procedure for other naris. Select one with greater air flow.	Tube passes more easily through naris that is more patent.

Steps	Rationale
8. Determine length of tube to be inserted and mark with tape.	Approximates depth of NG tube insertion.

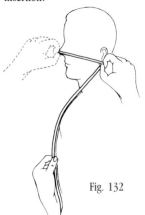

Fig. 132

Steps (continued)

8. (continued)
   a. Traditional method (Fig. 132): Measure distance from tip of nose to earlobe to xiphoid process to sternum.
   b. Hanson method: First mark 50 cm point on tube; then do traditional measurement. Tube insertion should be to midway point between 50 cm (25 inches) and traditional mark.

Large-Bore Intubation

Steps	Rationale
9. Prepare nasogastric tube for intubation:	
a. Plastic tubes should not be iced.	Tubes will become stiff and inflexible, causing trauma to mucous membranes.
10. Wash hands.	Reduces spread of microorganisms.
11. Put on clean gloves.	Protects nurse from transmission of microorganisms from gastric contents.
12. Lubricate nasogastric tube 10-20 cm.	Lubrication decreases friction between nasal mucous membrane and tube.
13. Alert client that insertion is to begin. Insert tube gently through nostril to back of throat (posterior nasopharynx). May cause client to gag. Aim back and down toward ear.	Natural contours facilitate passage of tube into gastrointestinal tract.

Steps	Rationale
14. Flex client's head toward chest after tube has passed through nasopharynx. Allow client to relax a moment.	Closes off glottis and reduces risk of tube entering trachea. Allows client to "catch breath" and remain calm.
15. Encourage client to swallow by giving small sips of water or ice chips when possible. Advance tube as client swallows. Rotate tube 180 degrees while inserting.	Swallowing facilitates passage of tube past oropharynx. Rotating tube decreases friction.
16. Emphasize need to mouth breath and swallow during procedure.	Helps facilitate passage of tube and alleviates client's fears during procedure.
17. Advance tube each time client swallows until desired length has been passed.	Reduces discomfort and trauma to client.
18. Do not force tube. When resistance is met or client starts to gag, choke, or become cyanotic, stop advancing tube and pull tube back. Check for position of tube in back of throat with tongue blade.	Tube may be coiled, kinked, in oropharynx or entering trachea.
19. Check placement of tube:	Proper position is essential before initiating feedings.
a. Attach a syringe to end of nasogastric tube. Place diaphragm of stethoscope over upper left quadrant of client's abdomen just below costal margin. Inject 10-20 ml of air while auscultating abdomen.) (Fig. 133)	Air entering stomach creates "whooshing" sound and confirms tube placement. Absence of sound indicates tip of tube is still in esophagus.

Fig. 133

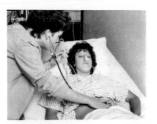

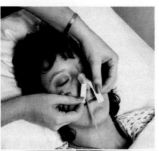

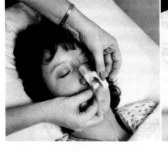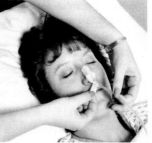

Fig. 134

Steps	Rationale
b. Aspirate gently to obtain gastric contents.	Another effective means for confirming tube placement. If tip is not in stomach, contents cannot be aspirated.
c. If tube is not in stomach, advance another 2.5-5 cm (1-2 inches) and again check position.	Tube must be in stomach to provide adequate decompression.

Steps	Rationale
20. Apply tincture of benzoin on tip of client's nose and tube. Allow to dry.	Helps tape adhere better.
21. Secure tube with tape and avoid pressure on naris.	Prevents trauma to nasal mucosa and permits client mobility.
a. Cut 10 cm (4 inches) long piece of tape. Split one end lengthwise 5 cm (2 in). Place other end of tape over bridge of patient's nose. Wrap 1.3 cm ($\frac{1}{2}$ inch) strips around tube as it exists nose (Fig. 134)	Prevents tissue necrosis to naris. Secures tape to nares.
b. Fasten end of nasogastric tube to client's gown by looping rubber band around tube in slip knot and pin to gown.	Reduces traction on the naris if tube moves. Provides slack to take if client moves.
22. Obtain x-ray of abdomen (tube must be radiopaque).	Determines placement of tube.
23. Administer oral hygiene frequently. Cleanse tubing at nostril.	Promotes client comfort and integrity of oral mucous membranes.
24. Remain and talk with client.	Decreases anxiety after tube insertion.

Small-Bore Intubation

9. Prepare NG tube for intubation:	
a. Plastic tubes should not be iced.	Tubes will become stiff and inflexible, causing trauma to mucous membranes.
b. Wash hands.	Reduces spread of microorganisms.
c. Inject 10 ml of water from 30 ml or larger luer-lok tip syringe into the tube.	Aids in guidewire or stylet insertion.

Steps	Rationale
d. Insert guidewire or stylet into tube, making certain it's securely positioned against weighted tip and that both luer-lok connections are snugly fitted together.	Promotes smooth passage of tube into GI tract. Improperly positioned stylet can induce serious trauma.
e. Dip weighted tip of tube into glass of water.	Activates lubricant to facilitate passage of tube into naris to GI tract.
10. Put on clean gloves.	Protects nurse from transmission of infection from GI contents.
11. Insert tube through nostril to back of throat (posterior nasopharynx). May cause client to gag. Aim back and down toward ear.	Natural contours facilitate passage of tube into GI tract.
12. Flex client's head toward chest after tube has passed through nasopharynx.	Closes off glottis and reduces risk of tube entering trachea.
13. Encourage client to swallow by giving small sips of water or ice chips when possible. Advance tube as client swallows. Rotate tube 180 degrees while inserting.	Swallowing facilitates passage of tube past oropharynx. Rotating tube decreases friction.
14. Emphasize need to mouth breath and swallow during the procedure.	Helps facilitate passage of tube and alleviates client's fears during the procedure.
15. Advance tube each time client swallows until desired length has been passed.	Reduces discomfort and trauma to client.
16. Do not force tube. When resistance is met or client starts to cough, choke, or become cyanotic, stop advancing the tube and pull	Tube may be coiled, kinked, or entering trachea.

Steps	Rationale
tube back. Check for position of tube in back of throat with tongue blade.	
17. Check placement of tube.	Proper position is essential before initiating feedings.
a. Aspirate GI contents with syringe.	Obtain recognizable GI contents to determine proper placement
b. Auscultate with stethoscope over left upper quadrant of abdomen and quickly inject 10 to 20 ml of air without resistance via syringe into tube.	Air (i.e., whooshing or gurgling sound) can be heard entering stomach. The reliability of this method can be disputed since the tube can be inadvertently placed in lungs, pharynx, or esophagus and transmit sound similar to that of air entering stomach. (Methany, 1988)
c. X-ray of tube placement needs to be done.	Determines that small-bore feeding tube is not in airway.
18. Apply tincture of benzoin on tip of client's nose and tube. Allow to dry.	Helps tape adhere better.
19. Secure tube with tape and avoid pressure on naris. Anchor tubing to client's gown when possible. (See Step 21, Large-bore intubation.)	Prevents trauma to nasal mucosa and permits client mobility.
20. Position client on right side when possible until radiological confirmation of correct placement has been verified.	Allow tube to pass small intestine (duodenum or jejunum).
21. Obtain x-ray of abdomen (tube must be radiopaque.)	Placement of tube is verified by x-ray examination.
22. Leave stylet in place until correct position is ensured by x-ray. Never attempt to reinsert partially or fully removed stylet while feeding tube is in place.	Guidewire or stylet may perforate GI tract, especially esophagus or nearby tissue and seriously injure the client.

Steps	Rationale
23. Remain and talk with client.	Decreases anxiety after tube insertion.
24. Administer oral hygiene frequently. Cleanse tubing at nostril.	Promotes client comfort and integrity of oral mucous membranes.
25. Remove gloves, dispose of equipment, wash hands.	Reduces transmission of microorganisms.
26. Record type of tube placed and client's tolerance to the procedure.	Documents the exact procedure.

Nurse Alert

Nasogastric tube placement can only be confirmed accurately by x-ray visualization and must be reassessed after the client's position changes or if severe coughing or vomiting develops. Verification determines that the tube is not displaced into the airway.

Client Teaching

Preprocedure instruction in relaxation and deep breathing exercises can help reduce client anxiety and promote cooperation during tube insertion.

Pediatric Considerations

Nasogastric tubes may be placed in infants or small children through either the mouth or the nares. The size of the tube varies with the size of the child and the viscosity of any solution being introduced (infants, 5 to 8 Fr; children, 10 to 14 Fr). Measurement is from (a) the bridge of the nose to the umbilicus or (b) the tip of the nose to the earlobe and then to the tip of the xiphoid process.

Geriatric Considerations

With aging there is a reduction in the amount of secretions produced by the stomach and intestinal tract.

Nasogastric Tube

Feedings

Initiating and maintaining nutrition

Enteral feeding is preferred over parenteral nutrition because it improves utilization of nutrients, is safer for clients, and is less expensive. Not all clients are able to be fed enterally, but if the gastrointestinal system is able to digest and absorb nutrients, it should be used. Indications for nasogastric tube feedings include clients who cannot eat, clients who will not eat, and clients who cannot maintain adequate oral nutrition (e.g., clients with cancer, sepsis, trauma, or clients who are comatose).

Potential Nursing Diagnoses

Pain related to placement of nasogastric tube
Altered nutrition: less than body requirements related to intolerance to tube feedings
Diarrhea related to initiation of tube feedings
Impaired gas exchange related to aspiration of gastric contents into respiratory tract

Equipment

Disposable gavage bag and tubing
60 ml catheter tip syringe (large-bore NG tube)
30 ml or larger luer-lok or tip syringe (small-bore NG tube)
Stethoscope
Prescribed tube feeding formula
Infusion pump (use pump designed for tube feedings)

Steps	Rationale
1. Wash hands.	Reduces transmission of micro-organisms.

Steps	Rationale
2. Auscultate for bowel sounds.	Bowel sounds indicate presence of peristalsis and ability of the GI tract to digest nutrients. When bowel sounds are absent, hold feeding and notify physician.
3. Verify physician's order for formula, rate, route, and frequency.	Tube feedings must be ordered by physician.
4. Prepare bag and tubing to administer formula: a. Connect tubing and bag. b. Fill bag and tubing with formula.	Tubing must be free of contamination to prevent bacterial growth. Placement of formula through tubing prevents excess air from entering gastrointestinal tract.
5. Explain procedure to client.	Reduces anxiety and increases cooperation.
6. Position client in high Fowler's position or elevate head of bed 30 degrees.	Reduces risk of aspiration.
7. Verify placement of NG tube. Large-bore intubation, Step 19. Small-bore intubation, Step 17.	Reduces risk of aspiration of gastric contents into the respiratory tract.
8. Initiate feeding: a. Bolus or intermittent method ■ Pinch proximal end of the feeding tube. ■ Attach syringe to end of tube and elevate to 18 inches above the client's head. ■ Fill syringe with formula. Allow syringe to empty gradually, refilling until pre-	Prevents air from entering client's stomach.

Steps	Rationale

scribed amount has been delivered to the client.

- If gavage bag is used, attach bag to the end of the feeding tube and raise bag 18 inches above client's head. Fill bag with prescribed amount of formula, allow bag to empty gradually over 30 min.

Gradual emptying of tube feeding by gravity from syringe or gavage bag reduces risk of diarrhea induced by bolus tube feedings.

b. Continuous drip method (Fig. 135)
- Hang gavage bag to IV pole.

Continuous feeding method is designed to deliver prescribed hourly rate of feeding. This method reduces risk of diarrhea. Clients who receive continuous drip feedings should have residuals checked every 4 hours.

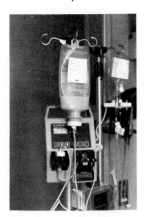

Fig. 135

- Connect end of bag to the proximal end of the feeding tube.
- Connect infusion pump and set rate.

9. When tube feedings are not being administered, clamp the proximal end of the feeding tube.

Prevents air from entering stomach between feedings.

Steps	Rationale
10. Administer water via feeding tube as ordered with or between feedings.	Provides client with source of water to help maintain fluid and electrolyte balance.
11. Rinse bag and tubing with warm water after all bolus feedings.	Rinsing bag and tube with warm water clears old tube feedings and prevents bacterial growth.
12. Advance tube feeding (see box).	Tube feedings should be advanced gradually to prevent diarrhea and gastric intolerance of formula.
13. Client remains in high Fowler's position or with head of bed elevated 30 degrees or more for 30 minutes after tube feeding. With continual feedings client should be in one of these positions throughout feeding.	Position uses gravity to assist in keeping formula in the GI tract. These positions reduce the client's risk of aspiration.
14. Record amount and type of feeding, verification of tube placement, patency of tube, client's response to feeding, and any adverse effects.	Documents status of tube feeding and client's response.

Nurse Alert

Some tube feedings are ordered over a 24-hour period, while others are ordered at intermittent periods. The physician determines the client's status and nutritional requirements when writing the nutritional orders. NG formulas should only be hung for 8 to 12 hours at room temperature.

Teaching Considerations

Teach the client and caregiver to keep tubing clamped between feedings and to give feedings with client in sitting position. If tolerated, client should remain upright for 30 minutes after feedings.

Pediatric Considerations

Intermittent feeding is preferred in infants because of possible perforation of stomach, nasal airway obstruction, ulceration, and irritation to mucous membrane.

Geriatric Considerations

Older adults may require a slower advance in tube feeding formula. The slower rate of formula advancement may assist in reducing the risk of diarrhea as a complication of NG tube feedings in this population.

Advance Tube Feeding

BOLUS

1. Advance concentration before increasing volume.
2. After client has tolerated desired concentration of feeding, advance volume over 24- to 48-hour period until maximum nutrient requirements are reached.
3. Aspirate before each feeding.
   a. Volume: 150 ml or more. Notify physician and withhold feeding. Check residual in 2 hours (if volume 150 ml or more again notify the physician so that client can be evaluated for delayed gastric emptying.
   b. Volume: less than 150 ml. Give tube feeding as ordered.

CONTINUOUS FEEDING

1. Advance concentration, then volume.
2. Initial infusion rate is usually 50 ml/hr.
3. After determining tolerance, advance in increments of 25 ml/hr daily until the necessary volume is reached or an infusion rate of 125 ml/hr.

Irrigating a Nasogastric Tube

Large-bore

A nasogastric tube is irrigated to maintain patency. If the distal tip of the tube rests against the stomach wall or if the tube becomes occluded with secretions, it must be irrigated. Obstruction of the tube can result in abdominal distention and possible vomiting. Nasogastric tube irrigations are routinely ordered when intermittent gastric suction is ordered.

Potential Nursing Diagnoses

Pain related to abdominal distention
Impaired skin integrity related to pressure from nasogastric tube against naris

Equipment

Soft or small bulb syringe or GU syringe
Normal saline, 30 ml
Emesis basin or irrigation tray
Towel
Facial tissues

Steps	Rationale
1. Wash hands.	Reduces transmission of microorganisms.
2. Check tube placement.	Prevents accidental entrance of irrigating solution into lungs.
▪ Attach syringe to end of nasogastric tube. Place diaphragm of stethoscope over upper left quadrant of client's abdomen just be-	Air entering stomach creates "whooshing" sound and confirms large-bore tube placement. Absence of sound indicates that tip of tube is still in esophagus.

Steps	Rationale
low costal margin. Inject 10-20 ml of air while auscultating abdomen.	
■ Aspirate gently to obtain gastric contents.	If tip is not in stomach, contents cannot be aspirated.
■ If tube is not in stomach, advance another 2.5-5 cm (1-2 inches) and check position.	Tubing must be in stomach to provide adequate decompression.
3. Draw up 30 ml of normal saline into bulb syringe.	Isotonic solution maintains osmotic pressure and minimizes loss of electrolytes from stomach.
4. Kink or clamp off tube proximal to connection site of drainage or suction apparatus. Disconnect suction tube and lay end on towel.	Prevents backflow of secretions and soiling of client's gown and bed linen.
5. Insert tip of irrigating syringe into end of nasogastric tube. Release clamp or kink in tube. Holding syringe with tip toward floor, inject saline slowly but evenly. (Do not force.)	Position of syringe prevents introduction of air into tubing. Air can cause distention. Fluid introduced under pressure can cause trauma.
6. If resistance occurs, check for kinks in tubing. Turn client on his side. Repeated resistance should be reported to physician.	Buildup of secretions will cause abdominal distention.
7. After instilling saline, immediately aspirate to withdraw fluid. Measure volume returned.	Stomach should remain empty. Fluid in stomach is measured as intake.
8. Reconnect nasogastric tube to drainage or suction. (If flow does not return, irrigation may be repeated.)	Reestablishes means of collecting drainage.

Steps	Rationale
9. Record irrigation procedure in nurse's notes. Mention specifically amount of normal saline instilled, amount and type of drainage returned, and client's tolerance.	Documents performance of procedure.

Nurse Alert

If a nasogastric tube continues to drain improperly after irrigation, the nurse must reposition it by advancing or withdrawing it slightly. Changes in the client's position or severe coughing or vomiting require reassessment of tube placement.

Client Teaching

Instruct the client to notify nursing personnel if the nasogastric tube becomes displaced or he feels nauseated. Nausea may be associated with abdominal distention due to improper draining of the tube. Irrigation of the tube may improve drainage and relieve the nausea.

Pediatric Considerations

Children are vulnerable to fluid and electrolyte imbalances associated with nasogastric suctioning. Therefore a meticulously accurate record of drainage and irrigating solution is essential. For irrigation an electrolyte solution is used to prevent further body depletion.

Geriatric Considerations

The older adult is vulnerable to fluid and electrolyte imbalances associated with nasogastric suctioning. Therefore accurate recording of drainage and irrigating solution is essential.

Clients with a nasogastric tube are NPO. An elderly person's oral mucosa can become dry and inflamed without thorough hygiene. Thus during nasogastric suctioning it is essential to keep the mucosa well hydrated.

Discontinuing a Nasogastric Tube

Large-bore and small-bore

Discontinuing a nasogastric tube is done when the client no longer needs gastric decompression, feeding, or lavage. Discontinuation of the nasogastric tube requires a physician's order.

Potential Nursing Diagnoses

Pain related to nasogastric tube
Impaired skin integrity related to NG tube against naris

Equipment

Facial tissue
Towel
Emesis basin
Toothbrush or sponge applicators for mouth care

Steps	Rationale
1. Wash hands.	Reduces transfer of microorganisms.
2. Place towel under client's chin.	Prevents contamination of bed or gown from gastric secretions.
3. Turn off suction and disconnect nasogastric tube from drainage bag. Remove tape from bridge of nose and remove pin from gown.	Tube should be free of connection when removed.
4. Explain procedure to client, reassuring him that removal is less distressing than insertion.	Minimizes client's anxiety.

Steps	Rationale
5. Hand client a facial tissue. Instruct him to take a deep breath and hold.	Airway may be temporarily obstructed during removal of tube. NOTE: Some clients may experience paroxysms of coughing during procedure.
6. Pull tube steadily and smoothly as client is holding his breath. (Do not pull too slowly or too rapidly.)	Reduces trauma to mucosa and minimizes client discomfort.
7. Dispose of tube and drainage equipment and wash hands.	Reduces transfer of microorganisms.
8. Clean client's nares and provide mouth care.	Promotes comfort. Nares often become excoriated.
9. Record procedure in nurse's notes. Mention specifically tube removal, final volume of secretions collected in drainage system, and client's response.	Timely recording accurately documents procedure.

Nurse Alert

After discontinuing a nasogastric tube the nurse should observe the client for abdominal distention, nausea, or vomiting. Any of these signs or symptoms could indicate the need for reinserting the tube.

DRESSINGS, BINDERS, AND BANDAGES

Changing a Dry Dressing

A dry dressing protects wounds with minimal drainage against microorganism contamination. The dressing can be simply a gauze pad that does not adhere to wound tissues and causes very little irritation. Or it can be a Telfa pad that, likewise, does not adhere to the incision or wound opening but allows drainage through the nonadherent surface to the softened gauze beneath.

As long as an incision or wound remains open, the application of a dry dressing requires sterile technique.

Potential Nursing Diagnoses

Impaired skin integrity related to surgical incision or traumatic wound

Pain related to incisional or traumatic wound

Impaired mobility related to pain

Equipment

Sterile dressing set or individual supplies of following:
  Sterile gloves
  Dressing set (scissors and forceps)
  Gauze dressings and pads
  Basin for antiseptic or cleaning solution
  Antiseptic ointment (optional)
Cleaning solution prescribed by physician
Normal saline or water
Disposable gloves
Tape, ties, or bandage as needed
Waterproof bag for disposal
Extra gauze dressings and Surgipads or ABD pads.
Bath blanket
Acetone (optional)

Steps	Rationale
1. Explain procedure to client by describing steps of wound care.	Relieves client anxiety and promotes understanding of healing process.
2. Assemble all necessary supplies at bedside table (do not yet open supplies).	Prevents chances of break in sterile technique by accidental omission of needed supplies.
3. Take disposable bag and make cuff at top. Place bag within reach of your work area.	Prevents accidental contamination of top of outer bag surface. Do not reach across sterile field to dispose of soiled dressing.
4. Close room or cubicle curtains or arrange partition around bed. Close any open windows.	Provides client privacy and reduces air currents that may transmit microorganisms.
5. Assist client to comfortable position and drape him with bath blanket to expose only wound site. Instruct client not to touch wound area or sterile supplies.	Sudden movement by client during dressing change can cause contamination of wound or supplies. Draping provides access to wound and minimizes unnecessary exposure.
6. Wash hands thoroughly.	Removes microorganisms resident on skin surface and reduces transmission of pathogens to exposed tissues.
7. Don clean disposable gloves and remove tape, ties, or bandage.	Gloves prevent transmission of infectious organisms from soiled dressings to your hands.
8. Remove tape by loosening end and pulling gently, parallel to skin and toward dressing. (If adhesive remains on skin, it may be removed with acetone.)	Reduces tension against suture line or wound edges.
9. With your gloved hand or forceps, lift dressings off, keeping soiled undersurface away from client's sight. NOTE: If drains are present, remove only one dressing at a time.	Appearance of drainage may upset client emotionally. Cautious removal of dressings prevents accidental withdrawal of drain.

Steps	Rationale
10. If dressing sticks to wound, loosen it by applying sterile saline or water.	Prevents disruption of epidermal surface.
11. Observe character and amount of drainage on dressings.	Provides estimate of drainage lost and assessment of wound's condition.
12. Dispose of soiled dressings in trash bag, avoiding contamination of bag's outer surface. Remove disposable gloves by pulling them inside out. Dispose of them properly.	Procedures reduce transmission of microorganisms to other persons.
13. Open sterile dressing tray or individually wrapped sterile supplies. Place on bedside table or at client's side on bed. Dressings, scissors, and forceps should remain in sterile tray or can be placed on open sterile drape used as a sterile field. Open bottle or packet of antiseptic solution and pour it into sterile basin or over sterile gauze. (Fig. 136)	Sterile dressings and supplies remain sterile while on or within a sterile surface. Preparation of all supplies prevents break in technique during actual dressing change.

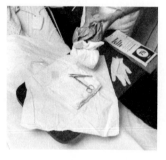

Fig. 136

Steps	Rationale
14. If sterile drape or gauze packages become wet from antiseptic solution, repeat preparation of supplies.	Fluids move through material by capillary action. Microorganisms travel from unsterile environment on table top or bed linen through dressing package to dressing itself.

Steps	Rationale
15. Don sterile gloves. (Fig. 137)	Allows you to handle sterile dressings, instruments, and solutions without contaminating them.

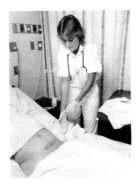

Fig. 137

| 16. Inspect wound. Note its condition, placement of drain, integrity of suture or skin closure, and character of drainage. (Palpate wound, if necessary, with portion of nondominant hand that will not touch sterile supplies.) (Fig. 138) | Determines state of wound healing. (Contact with skin surface or drainage contaminates glove.) |

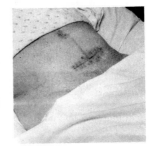

Fig. 138

| 17. Clean wound with prescribed antiseptic solution or normal saline. Grasp gauze moistened in solution with forceps. Use separate gauze for each cleaning stroke. Clean from least contaminated to most contaminated area. Move in progressive strokes away from incision or wound edges. | Use of forceps prevents contamination of gloved fingers. Direction of cleaning strokes prevents introduction of organisms into wound. |

Steps	Rationale
18. Use fresh gauze to dry wound or incision line. Swab in same manner as described in Step 17.	Reduces moisture at wound site, which eventually could harbor microorganisms.
19. Apply antiseptic ointment (if ordered), using same technique as for cleaning. Do not apply over drainage site.	Application directly to dressing or drainage site can occlude drainage.
20. Apply dry sterile dressings to incision or wound site. Apply dressings one at a time. (Fig. 139)	Prevents application of large bulky dressings that may impair client's movement and ensures proper coverage of entire wound.

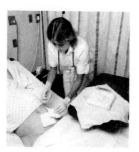

Fig. 139

■ Apply loose woven gauze (4 × 4) or Telfa as contact layer.	Promotes proper absorption of drainage.
■ If a drain is present, take scissors and cut 4 × 4 gauze square to fit around it.	Dressing around drain secures its placement and absorbs drainage.
■ Apply second layer of gauze as an absorbent layer.	
■ Apply thicker woven Surgipad or ABD pad. (Blue line down middle of pad marks outside surface.) (Fig. 140)	Protects wound from entrance of microorganisms.

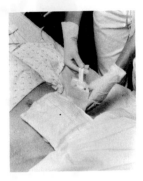
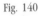

Fig. 140

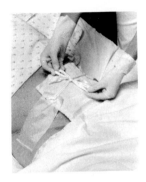

Fig. 141

Steps	Rationale
21. Use tape over dressing or secure with Montgomery ties, bandage, or binder. (Fig. 141)	Provides support to wound and ensures complete coverage with minimized exposure to microorganisms.
22. Remove gloves and dispose of them properly in container.	Reduces transmission of microorganisms.
23. Dispose of all supplies and help client return to comfortable position.	Clean environment enhances client comfort.
24. Wash hands.	Reduces microorganism transmission.
25. Record in nurse's notes observations of wound, dressing, and drainage. Document dressing change, including statement of client's response.	Accurate timely documentation notifies personnel of any changes in wound condition and status of client.

Nurse Alert

When removing or positioning the dressing, take care not to dislodge or pull on a drain. If the wound is dry and intact, healing may be optimized by exposing it to air. Contact the physician for an order to discontinue wound dressing.

Client Teaching

Clients often go home with a simple dry dressing in place. They, or their family, must be instructed in handwashing techniques, wound cleaning, and proper disposal of soiled dressings. It is not necessary to use sterile technique.

Pediatric Considerations

When a dressing is absolutely necessary in an infant or young child, the nurse should incorporate diversional activities into her care plan so the chances of the child's displacing the dressing will be minimized.

Geriatric Considerations

An elderly client's skin is normally inelastic and thin. Use special care, therefore, when removing tape.

Changing a Wet-to-Dry Dressing

A wet-to-dry dressing is the treatment of choice for wounds requiring debridement. The wet portion of the dressing effectively cleans an infected and necrotic wound. The moist gauze directly absorbs all exudate and wound debris. The dry outer layer helps pull moisture from the wound into the dressing by capillary action.

Potential Nursing Diagnoses

Potential for infection related to open wound
Impaired skin integrity related to wound infection
Pain related to open wound
Self-esteem disturbance related to wound drainage

Equipment

A sterile dressing set or individual supplies of following:
  Sterile gloves
  Sterile scissors and forceps
  Sterile drape (optional)
  Gauze dressings and fine-mesh 4 × 4 gauze pads
  Basin for antiseptic or cleaning solution
  Antiseptic ointment (optional)
Cleaning solution prescribed by physician
Normal saline or water
Disposable gloves
Tape, ties, or bandage as needed
Waterproof bag for disposal
Extra gauze dressings and Surgipads or ABD pads
Bath blanket
Acetone (optional)
Waterproof pad

Steps	Rationale
1. Explain procedure to client by describing steps of wound care.	Relieves client's anxiety and promotes understanding of healing process.
2. Assemble all necessary supplies at bedside table (do not yet open supplies).	Prevents chances of break in sterile technique by accidental omission of a needed supply.
3. Take disposable bag and make cuff at top. Place bag within reach of your work area.	Cuff prevents accidental contamination of top of outer bag surface. You should not reach across sterile field to dispose of soiled dressing.
4. Close room or cubicle curtains or arrange partition around bed. Close any open windows.	Provides client privacy and reduces air currents that may transmit microorganisms.
5. Assist client to comfortable position and drape him with bath blanket to expose only wound site. Instruct client not to touch wound area or sterile supplies.	Sudden movement by client during dressing change can cause contamination of wound or supplies. Draping provides access to wound and minimizes unnecessary exposure.
6. Wash hands thoroughly.	Removes microorganisms resident on skin surface and reduces transmission of pathogens to exposed tissues.
7. Place waterproof pad under client.	Prevents soiling of bed linen.
8. Don clean disposable gloves and remove tape, ties, or bandage.	Gloves prevent transmission of infectious organisms from soiled dressings to your hands.
9. Remove tape by loosening end and pulling gently, parallel to skin and toward dressing. (If adhesive remains on skin, it may be removed with acetone.)	Reduces tension against suture line or wound edges.

Steps	Rationale
10. With gloved hand or forceps, lift dressings off, keeping soiled undersurface away from client's sight. NOTE: If drains are present, remove only a layer at a time.	Appearance of drainage may upset client emotionally. Cautious removal of dressings prevents accidental withdrawal of drain.
11. If dressing adheres to underlying tissues, do not moisten it. Gently free the dressing from dried exudate. Warn client about pulling and possible discomfort.	Wet-to-dry dressing is designed to clean contaminated or infected wounds by debridement of necrotic tissue and exudate.
12. Observe character and amount of drainage on dressing.	Provides estimate of drainage lost and assessment of wound condition.
13. Dispose of soiled dressings in appropriate container, avoiding contamination of outer surface of container. Remove disposable gloves by pulling them inside out. Dispose of them properly.	Reduces transmission of microorganisms to other persons.
14. Prepare sterile dressing supplies. Pour the prescribed solution into a sterile basin and add fine-mesh gauze.	Contact layer of gauze must be totally moistened to increase dressing's absorptive abilities.
15. Don sterile gloves.	Allows you to handle sterile dressings, instruments, and solutions without contaminating them with microorganisms.
16. Inspect wound. Note its condition, placement of drain, integrity of sutures or skin closure, and character of drainage. (Palpate wound, if necessary, with portion of your nondominant hand that will not be touching sterile supplies.)	Determines state of wound healing. (Contact with skin surface or drainage contaminates glove.)

Steps	Rationale
17. Clean wound with pre-scribed antiseptic solution or normal saline. Grasp gauze moistened in solution with forceps. Use separate gauze square for each cleaning stroke. Clean from least contaminated to most contaminated area. Move in progressive strokes away from incision line or wound edges.	Use of forceps prevents contam-ination of your gloved fingers. Direction of cleaning prevents introduction of organisms into wound.
18. Apply moist fine-mesh gauze directly on wound surface. If wound is deep, gently pack it by first pick-ing up end of gauze with forceps. Gradually feed gauze into wound so all surfaces of wound are in contact with moist gauze. (Figs. 142 and 143)	Moist gauze absorbs drainage and adheres to debris. Pack gauze so it is evenly distributed within wound bed.

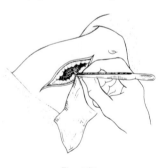

Fig. 142   Fig. 143

19. Apply dry sterile gauze (4× 4) over wet gauze.	Dry layer serves as absorbent layer to pull moisture from wound surface.
20. Cover with gauze, Surgi-pad, or ABD pad.	Gauze or pad protects wound from entrance of microorgan-isms.

Steps	Rationale
21. Apply tape over dressing or secure with Montgomery ties, bandage, or binder.	Provides support to wound and ensures complete coverage of wound to minimize exposure to microorganisms.
22. Assist client to comfortable position.	Enhances client's sense of well-being.
23. Wash hands.	Reduces transmission of micro-organisms.
24. Record in nurse's notes observations of wound, dressing, drainage, and client's response.	Accurate and timely documentation notifies personnel of any changes in wound condition and status of client.

Nurse Alert

Removal of the old dressing and reapplication of a new wet-to-dry dressing may cause the client pain. The nurse should administer an analgesic and time the dressing change to coincide with the drug's peak effect.

Client Teaching

A client is not usually discharged home while a wet-to-dry dressing is still required. He can be taught wound care in anticipation of use of a dry dressing at home.

Pediatric Considerations

It may be necessary to reinforce a wet-to-dry dressing with a gauze roll to prevent its accidental removal by an active toddler. Whenever possible, reinforce the dressing rather than restrain the child.

Geriatric Considerations

An elderly client's skin is normally thin and inelastic. Use special care, therefore, when removing tape.

Wound Irrigation

The purpose of wound irrigation is to remove exudate and debris from slow-healing wounds. It requires sterile technique and is particularly useful for open deep wounds, when access to all wound surfaces is limited. Wound irrigation can deliver heat to an affected area to promote healing or facilitate the application of local medications.

Potential Nursing Diagnoses

Impaired skin integrity related to open wound
Potential for infection related to open wound
Pain related to inflammation
Self-esteem disturbance related to wound drainage

Equipment

Sterile basin
Irrigating solution (200-500 ml as ordered) warmed to body temperature (32°-37° C or 90°-98.6°F)
Sterile irrigating syringe (sterile red rubber catheter as an attachment for deep wounds with small openings)
Clean basin to receive solution
Sterile dressing tray and supplies for dressing change
Waterproof pad
Lubricating jelly and tongue blade (optional)

Steps	Rationale
1. Explain procedure to client. Describe sensations to be felt during irrigation	Client's anxiety will be reduced through awareness of what procedure involves and sensations to be expected.

Steps	Rationale
2. Assemble supplies at bedside.	Prevents break in procedure.
3. Position client so irrigating solution will flow from upper end of wound into basin held below wound. (Fig. 144)	Fluid flows by gravity from least to most contaminated area.

Fig. 144

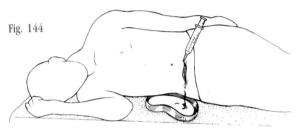

Steps	Rationale
4. Place waterproof pad under client.	Prevents soiling of bed linen.
5. Wash hands.	Reduces microorganism transmission.
6. Don clean disposable gloves and remove tape, ties, or bandage.	Gloves prevent transmission of infectious organisms from soiled dressings to your hands.
7. Remove tape by loosening end and pulling gently, parallel with skin and toward dressing. (If adhesive remains on the skin, it may be removed with acetone.)	Reduces tension against suture line or wound edges.
8. With your gloved hand or forceps, lift dressings off, keeping soiled undersurface away from client's sight. Remove one dressing layer at a time.	Appearance of drainage may upset client emotionally. Cautious removal of dressings prevents accidental withdrawal of drain.
9. If dressing sticks to wound, loosen it by applying sterile saline or water.	Prevents disruption of epidermal surface.

Steps	Rationale
10. Observe character and amount of drainage on dressings.	Provides estimate of drainage lost and assessment of wound's condition.
11. Dispose of soiled dressings in proper receptacle, avoiding contamination of receptacle's outer surface. Remove disposable gloves by pulling them inside out. Dispose of them properly.	Reduces transmission of micro-organisms to other persons.
12. Prepare sterile supplies. Open basin and pour in solution (volume varies depending on size of wound and extent of drainage). Open syringe. Prepare dressing tray. Don sterile gloves.	Prevents introduction of micro-organisms into wound.
13. Place clean basin against client's skin below incision or wound site.	Collects contaminated irrigating solution.
14. Draw up some solution into syringe. While holding syringe tip just above top of wound, irrigate slowly but continuously with enough force to flush away drainage and debris. Avoid sudden spurts or splashing of fluid. Irrigate pockets in wound.	Irrigation mechanically removes drainage and debris. Pockets or depressions in wound bed can easily trap debris.
15. Continue irrigating until solution draining into basin is clear.	Ensures that all debris has been removed.
16. With sterile gauze, dry off wound edges. Clean from least contaminated to most contaminated area. Move in progressive strokes away from incision line or wound edges.	Removes excess moisture, which can serve as medium for microorganism growth or as irritant to skin.

Steps	Rationale
17. Apply sterile dressing.	Sterile dressing prevents infection and promotes wound healing.
18. Assist client to comfortable position.	Promotes client comfort.
19. Dispose of equipment and wash hands.	Controls transfer of microorganisms.
20. Record in nurse's notes volume and type of solution, character of drainage, appearance of wound, and client's response.	Timely recording provides accurate documentation of therapy and progress of wound healing.

Nurse Alert

If drains are present, remove only one layer of dressing at a time so accidental withdrawal of a drain does not occur. Do not forcibly introduce irrigant into a wound pocket that is not visible. You could damage tissue.

Client Teaching

The client is not usually discharged home when irrigations are still necessary. However, instruct him regarding the procedure for wound irrigations so he can monitor the progress of his healing. In addition, early instruction helps him and his family prepare for discharge and any necessary home care.

Pediatric Considerations

If a child is unable to remain still during the procedure, it may be helpful for another nurse or the parent to use diversional activities such as reading, singing, or storytelling. Cautious use of restraints may be necessary.

Ear Irrigation

Irrigation of the auditory canal is performed to remove cerumen or a foreign object or to apply heat. The irrigating solution should be sterile to prevent transmission of microorganisms in the event of tympanic membrane rupture. The solution must be room temperature so it does not cause nausea or vertigo (severe dizziness). At home the client or family can be instructed in proper cleaning of the ear to reduce the need for further irrigation.

Potential Nursing Diagnoses

Potential for injury related to presence of foreign body in auditory canal

Sensory-perceptual alteration related to obstruction of ear canal

Pain related to inflammation of auditory canal

Equipment

Prescribed irrigating solution; volume depends on purpose: 200-500 ml at 37° C (98.6° F)

Sterile basin for solution

Soft or small bulb syringe

Curved emesis basin

Moisture-proof towel or pad

Cotton-tip applicators

Bath thermometer

Cotton balls

Steps	Rationale
1. Wash hands.	Reduces transmission of micro-organisms.

Steps	Rationale
2. Explain steps of procedure and warn client about sensations that might be experienced.	Relieves client's anxiety.
3. Assist client to either a side-lying or a sitting position with head tilted toward affected ear. Position emesis basin under ear. (Client may help hold basin.)	Irrigating solution will flow from auditory canal into basin.
4. Place towel over client's shoulder just under ear and emesis basin.	Prevents soiling of gown and bed linen.
5. Inspect auditory canal for any accumulation of cerumen or debris. Remove with cotton applicator and solution.	Prevents reentry of debris into canal during irrigation.
6. Check irrigating solution for proper temperature. Fill bulb syringe with appropriate volume.	Solution at body temperature minimizes onset of dizziness and discomfort.
7. Straighten auditory canal for introduction of solution. In infants, pull auricle (or pinna) down and back. In adults, pull auricle up and back.	Facilitates entrance and flow of irrigating solution.
8. With tip of syringe just above canal, irrigate gently by creating steady flow of solution against roof of canal.	Occlusion of canal with syringe causes pressure against tympanic membrane during irrigation. Flow of solution drains safely out of canal while loosening debris.
9. Continue irrigation until all debris has been removed or all solution has been used.	Purpose of irrigation may be to clean canal, instill antiseptics, or provide local heat.

Steps	Rationale
10. Assess client for onset of dizziness or nausea. Onset of symptoms may require temporary cessation of procedure.	Irritation of semicircular canals may cause dizziness and nausea.
11. Dry off auricle and apply cotton ball to auditory meatus.	Drying promotes client's comfort. Cotton ball collects excess drainage.
12. Position client on side of affected ear for 10 minutes.	Remaining solution in auditory canal will drain out.
13. Remove equipment and wash hands.	Controls transfer of microorganisms.
14. Return to client to assess character and amount of drainage and determine his level of comfort.	Enables you to evaluate client's tolerance of procedure.
15. Record in nurse's notes client's response to irrigation and note type, temperature, and volume of solution used and character of drainage.	Timely recording provides accurate documentation of client's response to procedure.
16. Return to client after 10 minutes to remove cotton ball and reassess drainage. Client may resume normal level of activity.	Increase in drainage or onset of pain may indicate injury to tympanic membrane.

Nurse Alert

Although the external auditory canal is not sterile, nevertheless you should use sterile drops and solutions in case the tympanic membrane (eardrum) is ruptured. Entrance of nonsterile solutions into the middle ear could result in infection. Never occlude the external auditory canal with the syringe. Forceful delivery of solution can damage the tympanic membrane.

Client Teaching

Family members as well as the client should be instructed not to force medication into an occluded auditory canal. Instilling medication or solution under pressure can injure the eardrum.

Pediatric Considerations

The auditory canal of infants and young children is straightened by grasping the pinna and pulling it gently downward and backward. Failure to straighten the canal properly may prevent medicinal solutions from reaching the deeper external ear structures.

Geriatric Considerations

The skin lining the auditory canal of an elderly person often becomes dry, flaky, and irritated. It is thus very important to be gentle when performing irrigations or cleanings of the ear in older clients.

Eye Irrigation

Eye irrigation is performed to relieve local inflammation of the conjunctiva, apply antiseptic solution, or flush out exudate or caustic or irritating solutions. It is a procedure commonly used in emergency situations when a foreign object or some other substance has entered the eye.

Potential Nursing Diagnoses

Sensory-perceptual alteration: visual related to inflammation and/
  or injury
Pain related to corneal or conjunctival injury
Anxiety related to visual impairment

Equipment

Prescribed irrigating solution; volume varies: 30-180 ml at 37° C
  (98.6° F) (For chemical flushing: tap water in volume to pro-
  vide continuous irrigation over 15 minutes)
Sterile basin for solution
Curved emesis basin
Waterproof pad or towel
Cotton balls
Soft bulb syringe or eye dropper
Disposable gloves (optional)

Steps	Rationale
1. Explain procedure fully to client. Explain that he will be allowed to close eye periodically and that no object will touch eye.	Relieves client's anxiety and improves his ability to cooperate.

Steps	Rationale
2. Assist client to lying position on side of affected eye. Turn his head toward affected eye.	Irrigating solution will flow from inner to outer canthus and into collecting basin.
3. Wash your hands.	Reduces number of microorganisms on skin surface.
4. Don disposable gloves (if client's eye is infected).	Prevents exposure of your hands to pathogens.
5. Place waterproof pad under client's face.	Prevents soiling of bed linen.
6. With cotton ball moistened in prescribed solution (or normal saline), gently clean lid margins and eyelashes. Clean from inner to outer canthus.	Minimizes transfer of debris from lids or lashes into eye during irrigation. Cleaning motion prevents entrance of drainage into nasolacrimal duct.
7. Place curved emesis basin just below client's cheek on side of affected eye.	Basin collects irrigating solution.
8. Fill irrigating syringe or eye dropper. Gently retract lower and upper eyelids (conjunctival sacs) by applying pressure to lower bony orbit and bony prominence beneath eyebrow. Do not apply pressure over eye.	Retraction minimizes blinking and exposes upper and lower conjunctival membranes for irrigation. Pressure on internal eye structures could cause permanent injury.
9. Hold irrigating syringe or dropper approximately 2.5 cm (1 inch) above inner canthus.	If dropper or syringe touches eye, there is risk of injury. Dropper or syringe becomes contaminated.
10. Ask client to look up. Gently irrigate by directing solution into lower conjunctival sac toward outer canthus. Use only enough force to remove secretions gently.	Flushing of conjunctival sac prevents exposure of sensitive cornea to solution. Fluid flows away from nasolacrimal duct, minimizing absorption of contaminated solution.

Steps	Rationale
11. Allow client to close his eye periodically, particularly if burning or excess blinking occurs. Encourage his cooperation.	Lid closure moves secretions from upper to lower conjunctival sac. Also promotes client's ability to relax during procedure.
12. Continue irrigation until all solution is used or secretions have been cleaned. (Remember: a 15-min irrigation is needed to flush chemicals.)	Serves to clean exudate, relieve inflammation, or flush caustic solution.
13. Dry eyelids and facial area with sterile cotton ball. Client may resume normal position.	Removes excess solution and provides for client's comfort.
14. Remove equipment and wash hands.	Reduces transfer of microorganisms.
15. Record in nurse's notes client's response to irrigation (burning, itching, pain) as well as volume and type of solution used, character of drainage, and appearance of conjunctiva.	Timely recording provides accurate documentation of client's response to procedure.

Nurse Alert

Be sure that a client's contact lenses are removed before beginning any irrigation. When caustic chemicals enter the eye, it is necessary to flush the eye continuously for at least 15 minutes. Continuous flushing prevents burning of the sensitive cornea. Do not apply pressure directly on the eye during irrigation. This could injure the eye.

Client Teaching

Clients can be taught to administer eye irrigations at home. However, they may need to use an eye cup, which should be practiced before it is attempted alone.

Pediatric Considerations

Young children are at risk of getting objects in their eyes accidentally during the normal course of play. The parent should act quickly, since a child's natural response is to begin rubbing his eye. It may be necessary to restrain a young child so the eye can be properly and thoroughly irrigated. The easiest technique is to have the child stand over a sink as the parent flushes the eye with tap water.

Geriatric Considerations

An elderly client may have reduced coordination of the hand or fingers and require assistance from an available family member or friend in administering the irrigation. If a client lives alone, he should try to perform the irrigation himself. Any delay could result in burns to the cornea.

Applying Binders

Abdominal, scultetus, and perineal T-binders

Binders provide support to large incisions. These incisions are vulnerable to tension or stress as the client moves or coughs. An abdominal binder is a rectangular piece of cotton or elasticized material that has either many tails attached to the two longer sides (as with the scultetus type or long extensions on each side to surround the abdomen (Fig. 145).

Perineal binders are designed for both male and female clients (Fig. 146). The male binder (also called a double T-binder) has two tails, which secure perineal or rectal dressings. The female binder (also called a T-binder) has one tail, which secures perineal or rectal dressings.

A properly secured binder provides support and comfort so the client can resume normal activities.

Potential Nursing Diagnoses

Pain related to incisional swelling
Impaired skin integrity related to open wound
Impaired physical mobility related to incisional pain
Ineffective breathing patterns related to incisional pain

Equipment
Binder: Abdominal, Scultetus, or Perineal

Steps	Rationale
1. Wash hands.	Reduces transmission of micro-organisms.

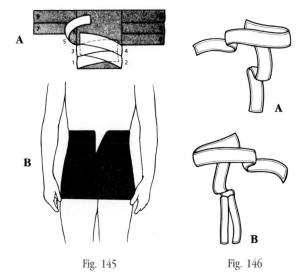

Fig. 145   Fig. 146

Steps	Rationale
2. Explain to client that binder serves to support abdominal incision and provides comfort.	Reduces client's anxiety.
3. Instruct client to roll onto one side while supporting abdominal incision and dressing firmly with hands.	Reduces pain.
4. Apply binder a. Abdominal or Scultetus ■ Place binder (fan folded) under client in same manner as when applying sheet for an occupied bed.	Allows client to roll over binder to ease positioning and centering.
■ Have client roll to opposite side. Unfold binder beneath him.	

Steps	Rationale
■ Position client supine over center of binder. Bottom edge of binder should be just above symphysis pubis, and top edge below costal margins.	Ensures that adequate pressure will be applied over wound. Also prevents interference with chest expansion.
■ Close the binder:	Firm even application provides optimal wound support and comfort.

Straight: Pull left end of binder toward center of client's abdomen. While keeping tension on left end, pull right end over left. Secure by smoothing Velcro edges together.

Scultetus: With your left hand, bring bottom tail at client's left side over toward center of abdomen. Keeping tension on tail, overlap it with bottom right tail. Repeat with each successive pair of tails, moving toward top of binder. Double the ends of tails back on themselves to prevent bulging or pressure areas. Be sure that each pair of tails overlaps pair below. Secure top pair with safety pin for each end. (Fig. 145)

Steps	Rationale
b. Perineal	
■ Provide perineal hygiene.	Ensure application of binder to clean skin.
■ Apply new perineal or rectal dressings according to physician's order.	Dressings to the perineal or rectal areas require frequent dressing changes, which assist in reducing the number of bacteria near the wound site.
■ Secure binder	
Female: Secure waist band. Bring vertical strip over perineal dressing and continue up and under center front, until vertical band can be secured to the waist band with safety pins.	Provides support to perineal muscles and organs.
Male: Secure waist band. Bring remaining vertical strips over dressing with each tail supporting one side of scrotum and proceeding upward on either side of penis. Continue until vertical tails can be secured to the waist band with safety pins.	
5. Assess client's comfort and ability to deep breathe and cough. Readjust as necessary.	Binders should exert pressure over abdomen, but should not impair chest expansion. Pernineal binders support perineal structures.
6. Wash hands.	Reduces transmission of microorganisms.
7. Record in nurse's notes application and client's tolerance.	Prompt documentation improves accuracy of record.

Nurse Alert

An abdominal binder should apply support to the abdominal structures but should never be so tight as to cause pain or impede deep breathing or coughing.

Client Teaching

Explanation of the procedure promotes client cooperation. In addition, teaching the client about why the binder is necessary can improve his mobility and his deep breathing and coughing.

Geriatric Considerations

An elderly person normally has, as a result of the aging process, reduced chest expansion and a diminished vital capacity. A binder should not restrict his ability to ventilate fully.

Applying Hot
Compresses

A hot moist compress is effective for improving circulation, re-
lieving edema, and promoting the consolidation and drainage of
pus. Because the compress is applied to an open wound, it must
be sterile.

Potential Nursing Diagnoses

Potential for infection related to an open wound
Pain related to incisional wound
Impaired physical mobility related to painful incision

Equipment

Prescribed solution warmed to proper temperature (approximately
   43°-46° C [110°-115° F])
Sterile gauze dressings
Sterile container for solution
Commercially prepared compresses (optional)
Sterile gloves
Petrolatum jelly
Sterile cotton swabs
Waterproof pad
Tape or ties
Dry bath towel
Water-flow or heating pad (optional)
Disposable gloves
Bath thermometer

Steps	Rationale
1. Explain procedure to client, including sensations to be felt (e.g., feeling of warmth and wetness). Explain precautions to prevent burning.	Improves client cooperation and lessens anxiety.
2. Assist client to comfortable position in proper body alignment.	Compress will remain in place for several minutes. Limited mobility in uncomfortable position can cause muscular stress.
3. Place waterproof pad under area to be treated.	Prevents soiling of bed linen.
4. Expose body part to be covered with compress. Drape rest of body with bath blanket.	Prevents unnecessary cooling and exposure of body part.
5. Wash hands.	Reduces transmission of infection.
6. Assemble equipment. Pour warmed solution in sterile container. (If using a portable heating source, keep solution warm. Commercially prepared compresses may remain under infrared lamp until just before use.) Open sterile packages and drop gauze into container to become immersed in solution. Turn electrical heating pad to correct temperature.	Compresses must retain warmth for therapeutic benefit.
7. Don disposable gloves. Remove any dressings covering wound. Dispose of gloves and dressings in proper receptacle.	Proper disposal prevents spread of microorganisms.
8. Assess condition of wound and surrounding skin.	Provides baseline for determining skin changes after compress application.

Steps	Rationale
9. Don sterile gloves.	Sterile touching sterile remains sterile.
10. Apply petrolatum jelly with a cotton swab to skin surrounding wound. Do not place jelly on areas of broken skin.	Protects skin from possible burns and maceration (softening).
11. Pick up one layer of immersed gauze and wring out any excess water.	Excess moisture macerates skin and increases risk of burns and infection.
12. Apply gauze lightly to open wound. Watch client's response and ask if he feels discomfort. In a few seconds, lift edge of gauze to assess skin for redness.	Skin is most sensitive to sudden change in temperature. Redness indicates a burn.
13. If client tolerates hot compress, pack gauze snugly against wound. Be sure that all wound surfaces are covered.	Packing of compress prevents rapid cooling from underlying air currents.
14. Wrap moist compress with dry bath towel. If necessary, pin or tie in place.	Insulates compress to prevent heat loss.
15. Change the hot compress every 5 minutes.	Prevents cooling, thus maintaining therapeutic benefit of compress.
16. (Optional) Apply waterflow or waterproof heating pad over towel. Keep it in place for desired duration of application (usually 20-30 min).	Provides constant temperature to compress.
17. Ask client periodically if there is any discomfort or burning sensation.	Continued exposure to heat can cause burning of skin.
18. Remove pad, towel, and compress. Assess wound and condition of surrounding skin.	Continued exposure to moisture will macerate skin.

Steps	Rationale
19. Replace sterile dressing.	Prevents entrance of microorganisms into wound site.
20. Dispose of equipment and wash hands.	
21. Record in nurse's notes type of application, solution, temperature of solution, duration of application, and condition of skin before and after procedure.	Accurate documentation protects you legally.

Nurse Alert

The nurse must use caution to avoid burning the client's skin. Because moisture conducts heat, the temperature setting on any device applied to a moist compress need not be as high as if the device is used for a dry application.

Client Teaching

Clients may frequently use compresses or heating devices in the house. Instruct them on ways to avoid burns: always time applications carefully to avoid overexposure; do not adjust the temperature of a heating pad to a high setting; do not lie directly on a heating device but instead apply it to the skin.

Pediatric Considerations

When applying a hot moist compress to a child, determine the need to restrain him so he does not contaminate the wound. If possible, you may use this time to cuddle and read to the child so as not to dislodge the compress.

Geriatric Considerations

Elderly persons frequently suffer a loss of or reduction in temperature sensation due to aging or chronic disease. Therefore, watch the client's skin condition carefully during heat application.

OXYGENATION

Postural Drainage

Postural drainage is the gravitational clearance of airway secretions from specific bronchial segments. It is achieved by assuming one or more of 10 different body positions. Each position drains a specific section of the tracheobronchial tree—the upper, middle, or lower lung field—into the trachea. Coughing or suctioning can then remove secretions from the trachea. The figures and list on the next pages show the bronchial area and the corresponding body posture for its drainage.

Potential Nursing Diagnoses

Ineffective airway clearance related to impaired cough
Ineffective breathing patterns related to decreased lung expansion
Impaired gas exchange related to retained airway secretions

Equipment

Pillows—two to three extra
Slant or tilt board (if drainage to be performed in home)
Facial tissues
Glass of water
Clear jar

Positions for Postural Drainage
Left and Right Upper Lobe Anterior Apical Bronchi

Have client sit in chair, leaning back against pillow.
(Figs. 147, 148)

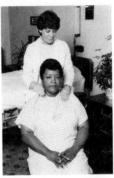

Fig. 147

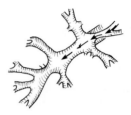

Fig. 148

Left and Right Upper Lobe Posterior Apical Bronchi

Have client sit in chair, leaning forward on pillow or table.
(Figs. 149, 150)

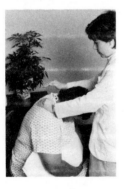

Fig. 149

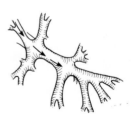

Fig. 150

Right and Left Anterior Upper Lobe Bronchi

Have client lie flat on back with small pillow under knees. (Figs. 151, 152)

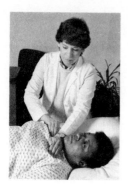

Fig. 151

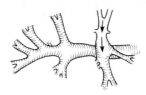

Fig. 152

Left Upper Lobe Lingual Bronchus

Have client lie on right side with arm over head in Trendelenburg position, with foot of bed raised 30 cm (12 inches). Place pillow behind back, and roll client one fourth turn onto pillow. (Figs. 153, 154)

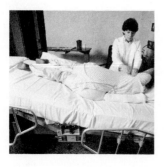

Fig. 153

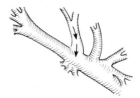

Fig. 154

Right Middle Lobe Bronchus

Have client lie on left side and raise foot of bed 30 cm (12 inches). Place pillow behind back and roll client one fourth turn onto pillow.
(Figs. 155, 156)

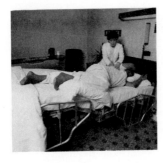

Fig. 155

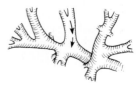

Fig. 156

Left and Right Anterior Lower Lobe Bronchi

Have client lie on back in Trendelenburg position, with foot of bed elevated 45-50 cm (18-20 inches). Have knees bent on pillow.
(Figs. 157, 158)

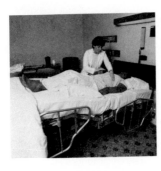

Fig. 157

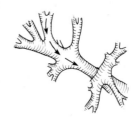

Fig. 158

Right Lower Lobe Lateral Bronchus

Have client lie on left side in Trendelenburg position with foot of bed raised 45-50 cm (18-20 inches).
(Figs. 159, 160)

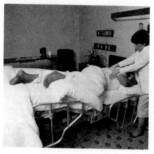
Fig. 159

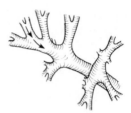
Fig. 160

Left Lower Lobe Lateral Bronchus

Have client lie on right side in Trendelenburg position with foot of bed raised 45-50 cm (18-20 inches).
(Figs. 161, 162)

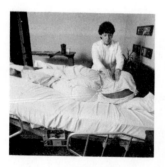
Fig. 161

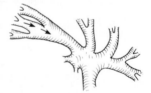
Fig. 162

Right and Left Lower Lobe Superior Bronchi

Have client lie flat on stomach with pillow under stomach.
(Figs. 163, 164)

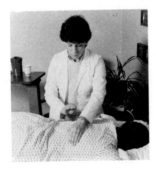

Fig. 163

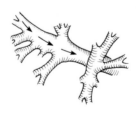

Fig. 164

Left and Right Posterior Basal Bronchi

Have client lie on stomach in Trendelenburg position with foot of
bed elevated 45-50 cm (18-20 inches).
(Figs. 165, 166)

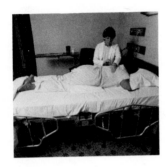

Fig. 165

Fig. 166

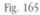

Steps	Rationale
1. Wash hands.	Reduces transmission of micro-organisms.
2. Select congested areas to be drained based on assessment of all lung fields, clinical data, and chest x-ray views.	To be effective, treatment must be individualized to treat specific areas involved.
3. Place client in position to drain congested areas. (First area selected may vary from client to client.) Help client assume position as needed. Teach client correct posture and arm and leg positioning. Place pillows for support and comfort.	Specific positions are selected to drain each area involved.
4. Have client maintain posture for 10-15 minutes.	In adults, draining each area takes time. In children, 3-5 minutes is sufficient.
5. During 10-15 minutes of drainage in this posture, perform chest percussion, vibration, and/or rib shaking over area being drained.	Provides mechanical forces that aid in mobilization of airway secretions.
6. After drainage in first posture, have client sit up and cough. Save expectorated secretions in clear container. If client cannot cough, suctioning should be performed.	Any secretions mobilized into central airways should be removed by cough and/or suctioning before client is placed in next drainage position. Coughing is most effective when client is sitting up and leaning forward.
7. Have client rest briefly if necessary.	Short rest periods between postures can prevent fatigue and help client to better tolerate therapy.
8. Have client take sips of water.	Keeping mouth moist aids in expectoration of secretions.

Steps	Rationale
9. Repeat Steps 3 to 8 until all congested areas selected have been drained. Each treatment should not exceed 30-60 minutes.	Postural drainage is used only to drain areas involved and is based on individual assessment.
10. Repeat chest assessment of all lung fields.	Allows you to assess need for further drainage or changes in drainage program.
11. Wash your hands.	Reduces transmission of micro-organisms.

Nurse Alert

Bronchospasm can be induced in some clients receiving postural drainage. It is caused by mobilization of secretions into the large central airways, which increases the work of breathing. To counteract the risk of bronchospasm, the nurse may ask the physician to start the client on bronchodilator therapy 20 minutes before postural drainage.

Client Teaching

The client and family should be taught how to assume postures at home. Some postures may need to be modified to meet individual needs. For example, the side-lying Trendelenburg position to drain the lateral lower lobes may have to be done with the client lying flat on his side or in a side-lying semi-Fowler position if he is very short of breath (dyspneic).

Pediatric Considerations

It is unrealistic to expect a child to cooperate fully in assuming all positions used for postural drainage. The nurse should set four to six positions as priority. More than six will frequently exceed the child's limit of tolerance.

Geriatric Considerations

Clients on antihypertensive medication may not be able to tolerate the postural changes required. The nurse must then modify the procedure to meet the client's tolerance and still clear his airways.

Oropharyngeal and Nasopharyngeal Suctioning

Oropharyngeal or nasopharyngeal suctioning is used when the client is able to cough effectively but is unable to clear secretions by expectorating or swallowing. It is frequently used after the client has coughed. Oropharyngeal and nasopharyngeal suction may also be appropriate in less responsive or comatose clients who require removal of oral secretions.

Potential Nursing Diagnoses

Ineffective airway clearance related to impaired cough reflex
Ineffective airway clearance related to immobility
Potential for infection related to pulmonary aspiration

Equipment

Portable or wall suction unit with connecting tubing and Y-connector if needed
Sterile catheter (12 or 16 French)
Sterile water or normal saline
Sterile gloves
Water soluble lubricant
Drape or towel to protect linen and client's bedclothes
Goggles

Steps	Rationale
1. Prepare equipment at bedside.	Allows smooth performance of procedure without interruption.
2. Wash hands and don goggles.	Reduces transmission of microorganisms.

Steps	Rationale
3. Explain to client how procedure will help clear airway and relieve some of his breathing problems. Explain that coughing, sneezing, or gagging is normal.	
4. Properly position client: • If conscious with a functional gag reflex—Place him in semi-Fowler position with head turned to one side for oral suctioning. Place him in semi-Fowler position with neck hyperextended for nasal suctioning.	Gag reflex helps prevent aspiration of gastrointestinal contents. Positioning head to one side or hyperextending neck promotes smooth insertion of catheter into oropharynx or nasopharynx respectively.
• If unconscious—Place him in lateral position facing you for oral or nasal suctioning.	Prevents client's tongue from obstructing airway, promotes drainage of pulmonary secretions, and prevents aspiration of gastrointestinal contents.
5. Place towel on pillow or under client's chin.	Soiling of bed linen or bed clothes from secretions is prevented. Towel can be discarded, reducing spread of bacteria.
6. Select proper suction pressure and the type of suction unit. For wall suction units this is 120-150 mm Hg in adults, 100-120 mm Hg in children, or 60-100 mm Hg in infants.	Assures safe negative pressure according to client's age. Excessive negative pressure can precipitate, injury to mucosa.
7. Pour sterile water or saline into sterile container.	Needed to lubricate catheter to decrease friction and promote smooth passage.
8. Put sterile glove on your dominant hand.	Maintains asepsis as catheter is passed into client's mouth or nose.

Steps	Rationale
9. Using your gloved hand, attach catheter to suction machine.	Sterility is maintained
10. Approximate the distance between client's earlobe and tip of nose and place thumb and forefinger of gloved hand at that point.	This distance ensures that suction catheter will remain in pharyngeal region. Insertion of catheter past this point places catheter in trachea.
11. Moisten catheter tip with sterile solution. Apply suction with tip in solution.	Moistening catheter tip reduces friction and eases insertion. Applying suction while catheter is in sterile solution ensures that suction equipment is functioning before catheter is inserted.
12. Suction ■ Oropharyngeal—Gently insert catheter into one side of client's mouth and guide it to oropharynx. Do not apply suction during insertion.	Stimulation of gag reflex is reduced.
■ Nasopharyngeal—Gently insert catheter into one naris. Guide it medially along floor of nasal cavity. Do not force catheter. If one naris is not patent, try other. Do not apply suction during insertion.	Catheter avoids nasal turbinates and enters more easily into nasopharynx. Risk of trauma to oral and nasal mucosa during catheter insertion is reduced.
13. Occlude suction port with your thumb. Gently rotate catheter as you withdraw it. Entire procedure should not take longer than 15 seconds.	Occlusion of suction port activates suction pressure. Suctioning is intermittently done as catheter is withdrawn. Rotation removes secretions from all surfaces of airway and prevents trauma from suction pressure on one area of airway. NOTE: Suctioning also removes air. Client's oxygen supply can be

Steps	Rationale
	severely reduced if procedure lasts longer than 15 seconds.
14. Flush catheter with sterile solution by placing it in solution and applying suction.	Removes secretions from catheter and lubricates it for next suctioning.
15. If client is not in respiratory distress, allow him to rest for 20-30 seconds before reinserting catheter.	Allows client opportunity to increase his oxygen intake.
16. If client is able, ask him to deep breathe and cough between suctions.	Promotes mobilization of secretions to upper airway, where they can be removed with catheter. If client is able to cough productively, further suctioning may not be needed so long as his airways are clear to auscultation.
17. If resuctioning is needed, repeat Steps 11 through 13.	
18. Suction secretions in mouth or under tongue after suctioning oropharynx or nasopharynx.	Sterile asepsis is maintained. Mouth should be suctioned only after sterile areas have been thoroughly suctioned.
19. Discard catheter by wrapping it around your gloved hand and pulling glove off around catheter.	Spread of bacteria from suction catheter is reduced.
20. Prepare equipment for next suctioning.	Ready access to suction equipment is provided, especially if the client is experiencing respiratory distress.
21. Record in nurse's notes amount, consistency, color, and odor of secretions as well as client's response to procedure.	Documents that procedure was completed.

Nurse Alert

If the client is unable to cough or has an artificial airway, orotracheal or nasotracheal suctioning is necessary.

Client Teaching

Clients who have undergone head and neck surgery (such as laryngectomy or neck dissection) often learn to self-administer oral suctioning while in the hospital. This can give them a sense of independence.

Pediatric Considerations

Children require smaller-diameter suction catheters. The newborn to 18-month-old child requires a 6 to 8 French, the 18-to-24-month old an 8 to 10 French, and the older child a 10 to 14 French.

Geriatric Considerations

Elderly clients with underlying cardiac or pulmonary disease may be able to tolerate only a 10-second period of suctioning. These clients are at greater risk of hypoxia-induced cardiac dysrhythmias.

Nasotracheal Suctioning

Nasotracheal suctioning involves the insertion of a small rubber tube into the client's naris and down to the trachea. The purpose of this procedure is to remove secretions from the client's airway and to stimulate the client to cough deeply. Secretions that are not removed from the airways increase the client's risk for infection and/or respiratory failure.

Potential Nursing Diagnoses

Ineffective airway clearance related to poor cough
Impaired gas exchange related to retained secretions

Equipment

Portable or wall suction unit with connecting tubing and Y-connector if needed
Sterile catheter (12 or 16 French)*
Sterile water or normal saline
Sterile cup*
Sterile gloves*
Water-soluble lubricant
Drape or towel to protect linen and client's bedclothes
Goggles

Steps	Rationale
1. Explain procedure to client.	Reduces anxiety and promotes cooperation.
2. Place client in semi- or high Fowler's position.	Position promotes maximum lung expansion.

*These materials are usually supplied in disposable suction kits.

Steps	Rationale
3. Wash hands.	Reduces transmission of micro-organisms.
4. Don goggles (Skill 6-3).	Protects the nurse from risk of transmission of blood-borne pathogens via droplet transmission.
5. If using suction kit:	
a. Open package. If sterile drape is available, place it across client's chest or use a towel.	Reduces transmission of micro-organisms.
b. Open suction catheter package. Do not allow suction catheter to touch any surface other than inside of its package.	Prepares catheter and reduces transmission of microorganisms. Maintains medical asepsis.
c. Unwrap or open sterile basin and place on bed-side table. Be careful not to touch inside of basin. Fill with about 100 ml sterile normal saline.	Saline is used to clean tubing after each suction pass.
6. Open lubricant. Squeeze onto open sterile catheter package without touching package.	Prepares lubricant while maintaining sterility. Water soluble lubricant is used to avoid lipoid aspiration pneumonia.
7. Apply sterile glove to each hand or apply nonsterile glove to nondominant hand and sterile glove to dominant hand.	Reduces transmission of micro-organisms and allows nurse to maintain sterility of suction catheter.
8. Pick up suction catheter with dominant hand without touching nonsterile surfaces. Pick up connecting tubing with nondominant hand. Secure catheter to tubing. (Fig. 167)	Maintains catheter sterility. Connects catheter to suction.

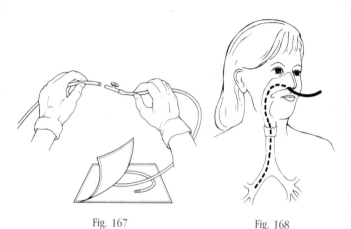

Fig. 167   Fig. 168

Steps	Rationale
9. Check that equipment is functioning properly by suctioning small amount of normal saline from basin.	Ensures equipment function. Lubricates internal catheter and tubing.
10. Coat distal 6-8 cm of catheter with water-soluble lubricant.	Lubricates catheter for easier insertion.
11. Remove oxygen delivery device, if applicable, with nondominant hand. Without applying suction, gently but quickly insert catheter with dominant thumb and forefinger into naris using slight downward slant or through mouth when client breathes in. Do not force through naris. (Fig. 168) a. Tracheal suctioning: in adults, insert catheter 20-24 cm; in older children, 14-20 cm; and in young children, and infants 8-14 cm.	Application of suction pressure while introducing catheter into trachea increases risk of damage to mucosa, as well as increased risk of hypoxia due to removal of inhaled oxygen present in airways. Epiglottis is open on inspiration and facilitates insertion into trachea. Client should cough. If client gags or becomes nauseated, catheter is most likely in esophagus.

Steps	Rationale

If resistance is felt after insertion of catheter for recommended distance, nurse has probably hit carina. Pull catheter back 1 cm before applying suction.

b. Positioning: in some instances turning client's head to right helps nurse suction left mainstem bronchus; turning head to left helps nurse suction right mainstem bronchus.

12. Apply intermittent suction for up to 10 seconds by placing and releasing non-dominant thumb over vent of catheter and slowly withdraw catheter while rotating it back and forth between dominant thumb and forefinger. Encourage client to cough. Replace oxygen device, if applicable.

Intermittent suction and rotation of catheter prevents injury to mucosa. If catheter "grabs" mucosa, remove thumb to release suction. Suctioning longer than 10 sec can cause cardiopulmonary compromise.

13. Rinse catheter and connecting tubing with normal saline until cleared.

Removes secretions from catheter.

14. Repeat Steps 10-12 as needed to clear pharynx or trachea of secretions. Allow adequate time between suction passes for ventilation.

Repeated passes with the suction catheter clear the airway of excessive secretions and promote oxygenation.

15. Monitor client's cardiopulmonary status between suction passes. Ask client to deep breath and cough.

Observe for alterations in cardiopulmonary status. Suctioning can induce hypoxia, dysrhythmias, and bronchospasm. Deep breathing reventilates and reoxygenates alveoli.

Steps	Rationale
16. When pharynx and trachea are sufficiently cleared of secretions, perform oral pharyngeal suctioning to clear mouth of secretions.	Removes upper airway secretions.
17. When suctioning is completed, roll catheter around fingers of dominant hand. Pull glove off inside out so that catheter remains coiled in glove. Pull off other glove in same way. Discard in appropriate receptacle. Turn off suction device.	Reduces transmission of microorganisms.
18. Remove towel, place in laundry.	Reduces transmission of microorganisms.
19. Reposition client.	Promotes comfort.
20. If indicated readjust oxygen to original level.	Prevents absorption atelectasis and oxygen toxicity.
21. Discard remainder of normal saline into appropriate receptacle. If basin is disposable, discard into appropriate receptacle. If basin is reusable, rinse it out and place it in soiled utility room.	Reduces transmission of microorganisms.
22. Wash hands.	Reduces transmission of microorganisms.
23. Place unopened suction kit on suction machine or at head of bed.	Provides immediate access to suction catheter.
24. Chart in nurses' notes respiratory assessments before and after suctioning; size of suction catheter used; duration of suctioning period; route(s) used to suction se-	Documents cardiopulmonary status, nursing care, expected and unexpected outcomes, and provides baseline for future assessment.

Steps	Rationale

cretions obtained; odor,
amount, color, consistency
of secretions; frequency of
suctioning; client's tolerance of procedure; amount
of negative suction pressure
used.

Nurse Alert

Clients with a history of deviated septum or facial trauma may require placement of nasal airway before nasal tracheal suctioning is attempted. Frequent nasotracheal suctioning may result in trauma to the nasal mucosa and bloody returns from the suction catheter.

Client Teaching

Clients who have undergone head and neck surgery (such as laryngectomy or neck dissection) often learn to self-administer oral suctioning while in the hospital. This can give them a sense of independence.

Pediatric Considerations

Children require smaller-diameter suction catheters. The newborn to 18-month-old child requires a 6 to 8 French, the 18-to-24-month old an 8 to 10 French, and the older child a 10 to 14 French.

Geriatric Considerations

Elderly clients with underlying cardiac or pulmonary disease may be able to tolerate only a 10-second period of suctioning. These clients are at greater risk of hypoxia-induced cardiac dysrhythmias.

Tracheal Suctioning

Tracheal suctioning involves the insertion of a suction catheter into the client's tracheal artificial airway. Tracheal suctioning maintains airway patency, facilitates removal of airway secretions, and stimulates a deep cough. In the acute health care environment tracheal suctioning is a sterile process. In the home setting the client may be instructed to use a clean suction technique as long as there are no signs of infection.

Potential Nursing Diagnoses

Ineffective airway clearance related to impaired cough
Potential for infection related to retained secretions
Impaired gas exchange related to retained airway secretions

Equipment

Bedside table
Suction catheter of appropriate size (see box)
Water-soluble lubricant
2 sterile gloves or 1 sterile and 1 nonsterile glove
Sterile basin
Approximately 100 ml sterile normal saline
Clean towel or sterile drape from kit
Portable or wall suction apparatus
6 ft of connecting tubing
Sterile suction kit can be used, if available (be sure all listed items not in kit are assembled)

APPROPRIATE CATHETER SIZE FOR CLIENT

Newborn	6-8 Fr
Infant to 18 mo	6-8 Fr
18 mo	8-10 Fr
24 mo	10 Fr
2-4 yr	10-12 Fr
4-7 yr	12 Fr
7-10 yr	12-14 Fr
10-12 yr	14 Fr
Adults	12-16 Fr

VACUUM SETTING

	Wall:	Portable:
Infants	60-100 mm Hg	3-5 inches Hg
Children	100-120 mm Hg	5-10 inches Hg
Adults	120-150 mm Hg	7-15 inches Hg

Steps	Rationale
1. Prepare client:	
a. Explain procedure and client's participation.	Encourages cooperation, minimizes risks, reduces anxiety.
b. Explain importance of coughing during procedure. Practice now, if able.	Facilitates secretion removal and may reduce frequency of future suctioning.
c. Assist client to assume position comfortable for nurse and client, usually semi-Fowler's or Fowler's. If unconscious, place in side-lying position.	Promotes client comfort; prevents muscle strain. Promotes maximum lung expansion and deep breathing. Also reduces risk of aspiration.
d. Place towel across client's chest.	Reduces transmission of microorganisms.
2. Wash hands.	Reduces transmission of microorganisms.
3. Turn suction device on and set vacuum regulator to appropriate negative pressure (see box).	Excessive negative pressure damages tracheal mucosa and can induce greater hypoxia.

Steps	Rationale
4. Connect one end of connecting tubing to suction machine and place other end in convenient location.	Prepares suction apparatus.
5. If using sterile suction kit:	
a. Open package. If sterile drape is available, place it across client's chest.	Prevents contamination of clothing.
b. Open suction catheter package. Do not allow suction catheter to touch any nonsterile surface.	Prepares catheter and prevents transmission of microorganisms.
c. Unwrap or open sterile basin and place on bedside table. Be careful not to touch inside basin. Fill with about 100 ml sterile normal saline.	Prepares catheter and prevents transmission of microorganisms.
6. If indicated, open lubricant. Squeeze onto sterile catheter package without touching package.	Prepares lubricant for use while maintaining sterility.
7. Apply one sterile glove to each hand or apply nonsterile glove to nondominant hand and sterile glove to dominant hand.	Reduces transmission of microorganisms and allows nurse to maintain sterility of suction catheter.
8. Pick up suction catheter with dominant hand without touching nonsterile surfaces. Pick up connecting tubing with nondominant hand. Secure catheter to tubing.	Maintains catheter sterility.
9. Check that equipment is functioning properly by suctioning small amount of saline from basin.	Ensures equipment function; lubricates catheter and tubing.

Steps	Rationale
10. Coat distal 6-8 cm of catheter with water-soluble lubricant. In some situations catheter is lubricated only with normal saline. Nursing assessment indicates need for lubrication.	Promotes easier catheter insertion. If lubricant is needed, it must be water soluble to prevent petroleum-based aspiration pneumonia. Excessive lubricant can adhere to artificial airway.
11. Remove oxygen or humidity delivery device with nondominant hand.	Exposes artificial airway.
12. Hyperinflate and/or oxygenate client before suctioning, using manual resuscitation (AMBU) bag or sigh mechanism on mechanical ventilator.	Hyperinflation decreases atelectasis caused by negative pressure. Preoxygenation converts large proportion of resident lung gas to 100% O_2 to offset amount used in metabolic consumption while ventilator or oxygenation is interrupted, as well as to offset volume lost out of suction catheter (Luce, 1984).
13. Without applying suction, gently but quickly insert catheter with dominant thumb and forefinger into artificial airway (best to time catheter insertion with inspiration).	Places catheter in tracheobronchial tree. Application of suction pressure while introducing catheter into trachea increases risk of damage to tracheal mucosa, as well as increased hypoxia due to removal of inhaled oxygen present in airways.
14. Insert catheter until resistance is met, then pull back 1 cm.	Stimulates cough and removes catheter from mucosal wall.
15. Apply intermittent suction by placing and releasing nondominant thumb over vent of catheter and slowly withdraw catheter while rotating it back and forth between dominant thumb and forefinger. Encourage client to cough.	Intermittent suction and rotation of catheter prevents injury to tracheal mucosal lining. If catheter "grabs" mucosa, remove thumb to release suction.

Steps	Rationale
16. Replace oxygen delivery device. Encourage client to deep breathe.	Reoxygenates and reexpands alveoli. Suctioning can cause hypoxemia and atelectasis.
17. Rinse catheter and connecting tubing with normal saline until clear. Use continuous suction.	Removes catheter secretions. Secretions left in tubing decrease suction and provide environment for microorganism growth.
18. Repeat Steps 12-17 as needed to clear secretions. Allow adequate time (at least 1 full min) between suction passes for ventilation and reoxygenation.	Repeated passes with suction catheter clear airway of excessive secretions and promote improved oxygenation.
19. Assess client's cardiopulmonary status between suction passes.	Suctioning can induce dysrhythmias, hypoxia, and bronchospasm.
20. When artificial airway and tracheobronchial tree are sufficiently cleared of secretions, perform nasal and oral pharyngeal suctioning to clear upper airway of secretions. After nasal and oral pharyngeal suctioning are performed, catheter is contaminated; do not reinsert into ET or TT.	Removes upper airway secretions. Upper airway is considered "clean" while lower airway is considered "sterile." Therefore, same catheter can be used to suction from sterile to clean areas, but not from clean to sterile areas.
21. Disconnect catheter from connecting tubing. Roll catheter around fingers of dominant hand. Pull glove off inside out so that catheter remains in glove. Pull off other glove in same way. Discard into appropriate receptacle. Turn off suction device.	Reduces transmission of microorganisms.

Steps	Rationale
22. Remove towel and place in laundry, or remove drape and discard in appropriate receptacle.	Reduces transmission of microorganisms.
23. Reposition client.	Promotes comfort. Sims' position encourages drainage and reduces risk of aspiration.
24. Discard remainder of normal saline into appropriate receptacle. If basin is disposable, discard into appropriate receptacle. If basin is reusable, place it in soiled utility room.	Reduces transmission of microorganisms.
25. Wash hands.	Reduces transmission of microorganisms.
26. Place unopened suction kit on suction machine or at head of bed.	Provides immediate access to suction catheter.
27. Record respiratory assessment before and after suctioning, size of suction catheter used, duration of suction procedure, secretions, and client's tolerance to procedure.	Documents cardiopulmonary status, nursing care given, and provides baseline for further assessments.

Nurse Alert

When a client has a tracheostomy tube, there is a loss of upper airway function that includes warming, filtering, humidifying. When thick, sticky secretions are present, assess hydration and monitor for the presence of infection.

Teaching Considerations

Clients in the home care environment need to be taught how to safely suction the tracheostomy tube. In addition, these clients must know when to used clean or sterile suction techniques and when to notify their physician.

Tracheostomy Care

Clients who have tracheostomy tubes require specialized nursing care to manage the tracheostomy tube itself and the stoma in the client's neck. The stoma provides the access for the tracheostomy tube in the client's tracheal airway.

Potential Nursing Diagnoses

Potential for infection related to crustations around tracheal stoma

Body-image disturbance related to artificial airway

Impaired skin integrity related to tracheostomy incision

Equipment (Fig. 169)

Bedside table
Towel
Tracheostomy suction supplies
Sterile tracheostomy care kit, if available (be sure all supplies listed that are not available in kit are collected)
Sterile 4 × 4 gauze—3 pkg
Hydrogen peroxide
Normal saline
Sterile cotton-tipped swabs
Sterile tracheostomy dressing (precut and sewn surgical dressing)
Sterile basin
Small sterile brush
Roll of twill tape or tracheostomy ties
Scissors
2 sterile gloves

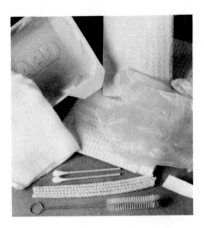

Fig. 169

Steps	Rationale
1. Have another nurse assist in this procedure (optional).	Prevents accidental extubation of tracheostomy tube.
2. Prepare client: a. Explain procedure and client's participation.	Encourages cooperation, minimizes risks, and reduces anxiety.
b. Assist client to position comfortable for both nurse and client (usually supine or semi-Fowler's).	Promotes client comfort, prevents nurse muscle strain.
c. Place towel across client's chest.	Reduces transmission of microorganisms.
3. Wash hands.	Reduces transmission of microorganisms.
4. Administer tracheostomy suctioning. Before removing gloves, remove soiled tracheostomy dressing and discard in glove with coiled catheter.	Removes secretions so as not to occlude outer cannula while inner cannula is removed.

Steps	Rationale
5. While client is replenishing oxygen stores, prepare equipment on bedside table. Open sterile tracheostomy kit. Open three 4 × 4 gauze packages aseptically and pour normal saline on one package and hydrogen peroxide on another. Leave third package dry. Open two cotton-tipped swab packages and pour normal saline on one package and hydrogen peroxide on the other. Open sterile tracheostomy dressing package. Unwrap sterile basin and pour about 1.8 ml (0.75 in) in hydrogen peroxide into it. Open small sterile brush package and place aseptically into sterile basin. If using large roll of twill tape, cut appropriate length of tape and lay aside in dry area. Do not recap hydrogen peroxide and normal saline.	Prepares equipment and allows for smooth organized completion of tracheostomy care.
6. Apply gloves. Keep dominant hand sterile throughout procedure. (For TT with inner cannula, complete Steps 7-19. For TT with no inner cannula or Kistner button, complete Steps 11-19).	Reduces transmission of microorganisms.
7. Remove oxygen source and then inner cannula with nondominant hand. Drop inner cannula into hydrogen peroxide basin.	Removes inner cannula for cleaning. Hydrogen peroxide loosens secretions from inner cannula.

Steps	Rationale
8. Place tracheostomy collar oxygen source over outer cannula. Place T-tube (Briggs) and ventilator oxygen sources over or near outer cannula.	Maintains supply of oxygen to client.
NOTE: T-tube and ventilator oxygen devices cannot be attached to all outer cannulas when the inner cannula is removed.	
9. To prevent oxygen desaturation in affected clients, quickly pick up inner cannula and use small brush to remove secretions inside and outside cannula.	Tracheostomy brush provides mechanical force to remove thick or dried secretions.
10. Hold inner cannula over basin and rinse with normal saline, using nondominant hand to pour normal saline.	Removes secretions and hydrogen peroxide from inner cannula.
11. Replace inner cannula and secure "locking" mechanism. Reapply T-tube (Briggs) and ventilator oxygen sources.	Secures inner cannula and reestablishes oxygen supply.
12. Using hydrogen peroxide-prepared cotton-tipped swabs and 4 × 4 gauze, clean exposed outer cannula surfaces and stoma under faceplate extending 4-8 cm (2-4 in) in all directions from stoma. Clean in circular motion from stoma site outward using dominant hand to handle sterile supplies.	Aseptically removes secretions from stoma site.

Steps	Rationale
13. Using normal saline-prepared cotton-tipped swabs and 4 × 4 gauze, rinse exposed outer cannula surfaces and stoma under faceplate extending 4-8 cm (2-4 in) in all directions from stoma. Rinse in circular motion from stoma site outward using dominant hand to handle sterile supplies.	Rinses hydrogen peroxide from surfaces.
14. Using dry 4 × 4 gauze, pat lightly at skin and exposed outer cannula surfaces.	Dry surfaces prohibit formation of moist environment for microorganism growth and skin excoriation.
15. Instruct assistant, if available, to securely hold TT in place. With assistant holding TT, cut ties. Assistant must *not* release hold on tracheostomy tube until new ties are firmly tied. If no assistant, do not cut old ties until new ties are in place and securely tied:	Promotes hygiene, reduces transmission of microorganisms. Secure TT.
a. Cut a length of twill tape long enough to go around client's neck two times; cut ends on diagonal.	Cutting ends of tie on diagonal aids in inserting tie through eyelet.
b. Insert one end of tie through faceplate eyelet and pull ends even.	
c. Slide both ends of tie behind head and around neck to other eyelet and insert one tie through second eyelet.	
d. Pull snugly.	

Steps	Rationale
e. Tie ends securely in double square knot allowing space for only one finger in tie.	One finger slack prevents ties from being too tight when tracheostomy dressing is in place.
16. Insert fresh tracheostomy dressing under clean ties and faceplate. (Fig. 170)	Absorbs drainage.

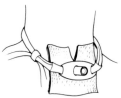

Fig. 170

17. Remove gloves and discard in appropriate receptacle with soiled tracheostomy ties.	Reduces transmission of micro-organisms.
18. Replace cap on hydrogen peroxide and normal saline bottles. Store reusable liquids and unused supplies in appropriate place.	Once opened, normal saline can be considered free of bacteria for 24 hours, after which it should be discarded.
19. Position client comfortably and assess respiratory status.	Promotes comfort. Some clients may require posttracheostomy care suctioning.
20. Wash hands.	Reduces transmission of micro-organisms.
21. Record assessment of client's respiratory status and status of skin around stoma, frequency of care, and tolerance to care.	Documents cardiopulmonary and tracheostomy site status, nursing care, and client's response to procedure.

Nurse Alert

There are alternate methods to apply tracheostomy ties. The one presented here is the safest and easiest to master. Commercial products that use Velcro and similar fastening devices are available in some institutions. Clients with new tracheostomy frequently have blood secretions for 2 to 3 days after procedure or for 24 hours after each tracheostomy tube change.

Do not cut 4 × 4 gauze. Loose strings that enter stoma can cause infection and irritation.

Teaching Considerations

Clients who are sent home with a tracheostomy tube must be taught how to safely and correctly complete tracheostomy care. Even when the client is able to complete the care, a family member or close friend should also learn the procedure in the event that the client is unable to complete the procedure.

Care of Chest Tubes

Trauma, disease, or surgery can result in air or fluid leaking into the intrapleural space. Small leaks are absorbed spontaneously. Closed chest drainage systems restore optimal lung expansion and promote the drainage of fluid and blood from the pleural space.

Potential Nursing Diagnoses

Impaired gas exchange related to limited lung expansion
Pain related to collapsed lung or chest tube insertion
Anxiety related to respiratory distress

Equipment

Chest tube insertion tray
Chest tube
Povidone-Iodine (Betadine)
Lidocaine
Sutures
Requested drainage system (one-, two- or three-bottle system or a disposable commercial system) (Fig. 171)
Sterile water or saline
Drainage tubing
Sterile gloves
Adhesive tape (0.5-1 inch)
Two shodded hemostats for each chest tube
Dressing materials: sterile wick, noncotton-filled 4 × 4 gauze pads, petroleum gauze and ABDs or combination dressings, wide adhesive tape or elastoplast

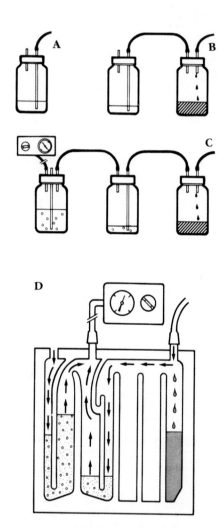

Fig. 171
Three types of chest tube bottle systems. **A,** One-bottle system. **B,** Two-bottle system. **C,** Three-bottle system with suction. **D,** Disposable, commercial chest drainage system.

Steps	Rationale
1. Assess client's cardiopulmonary status, observe for respiratory status, use of accessory muscles, color, pain, anxiety, and vital signs.	Provides continual data about client's status prior to, during, and after the chest tube procedure.
2. Review physician's role and responsibilities for chest tube placement (Table 4).	Helps differentiate doctor and nurse roles so that the nurse can function more effectively.
3. Explain procedure to client.	Reduces anxiety and promotes patient cooperation.
4. Wash hands.	Reduces transmission of microorganism.
5. Set up the prescribed drainage system:	Provides prescribed closed-drainage system.
a. One-bottle system:	
■ Obtain a vented water-seal chest tube drainage bottle and remove space, cover from vent.	Vent allows air to be expressed from the intrapleural space during each expiration, until the lung is reexpanded (Erickson, 1981a). Prevents formation of positive pressure in the intrapleural space and drainage system, which would impede drainage.
■ Pour sterile water or saline into bottle so that straw tip is submerged 2 cm (1 in).	Produces water seal and blocks air from reentering intrapleural space. Deeper submersion of the straw tip impedes drainage.
■ Assess system to ensure that all connections are airtight and the air vent is open.	Prevents atmospheric air from leaking into the system and the client's intrapleural space. Fluid and/or air will stop draining if negative pressure is not maintained in the system.
■ Tape all connections in a spiral manner.	Helps maintain an airtight seal. Allows visualization of drainage in the tubing.

Table 4   Physician's role and responsibility in chest tube placement

1. Explain purpose, procedure, and possible complications to the client.	Provides informed consent.
2. Wash hands. Cleanse chest wall with antiseptic.	Reduces transmission of microorganisms.
3. Don mask and gloves.	Maintains surgical asepsis.
4. Drape area of chest tube insertion with sterile towels.	Maintains surgical asepsis.
5. Inject local anesthesia and allow time to take effect.	Decreases pain during procedure.
6. Use blunt or sharp dissection to create incision in the skin and chest wall.	Opens chest for insertion of chest tube. A trochar is outdated and increases risk of tissue damage.
7. Thread a clamped chest tube through the incision. Physician clamps chest tube until system is connected to water seal.	Inserts chest tube into the intrapleural space. Clamping prevents entry of atmospheric air into the chest and worsening of the pneumothorax.
8. Suture chest tube in place, if suturing is policy or physician preference.	Secures chest tube in place.
9. Cover the chest insertion site with a large, sterile occlusive pressure dressing.	Holds chest tube in place and prevents air leakage around the tube to prevent additional atmospheric air from entering the intrapleural space.
10. Remove connector cover from client's end of chest drainage tubing, using sterile technique. Secure drainage tubing to the chest tube and drainage system.	Physician is responsible for making certain that the system is set up properly, the proper amount of water is in the water-seal, the dressing is secure, and the chest tube is securely connected to the drainage system.

Table 4   Physician's role and responsibility in chest tube placement—cont'd

11. Connect system to suction or supervise a nurse connecting it to suction, if suction is to be used.	The physician is responsible for determining and checking the amount of water that is to be added to the suction-control bottle/chamber and prescribing the suction setting.
12. Unclamp the chest tube.	Connects chest tube to the water-seal drainage and suction, thus promoting drainage of fluid or air from the intrapleural space and allowing the lung to reexpand.
13. Order and review chest x-ray.	Verifies correct chest tube placement.

Steps	Rationale
▪ If, during an emergency situation, a one-bottle system is used to drain fluid, place calibrated adhesive tape on side of the bottle.	Permits timely and efficient account of amount of drainage from the chest tube. Drainage is marked at specified periods of time and documented on the nurses' notes and I & O sheet.
▪ Observe depth of the water-seal tip below the drainage level.	The deeper the water-seal straw tip is submerged beyond 2 cm, the greater the resistance to drainage.
b. Two-bottle system:	
▪ Obtain a drainage collection bottle.	Collects intrapleural fluids drained by gravity into the first bottle without disturbing the water-seal.
▪ Obtain a vented water-seal bottle.	Blocks air from entering the intrapleural space. Vent allows air to escape from the water-seal bottle into the atmosphere.

Steps	Rationale
■ Pour sterile saline or water into water-seal bottle so the straw tip is submerged 2 cm (1 in).	Establishes water-seal, preventing air from reentering intrapleural space on inspiration.
■ Obtain connector tubing. Connect chest tube to the first (drainage) bottle rod. The second rod of this bottle is then connected to the water-seal straw. A final rod in the water-seal bottle is left open to air.	Tubing connects the chest tube to the drainage system. Drainage passes through tubing and into drainage bottle. Air, equal to the amount of drainage, passes from the drainage bottle through the water-seal bottle and into the atmosphere through the air vent.
■ Assess system to ensure that all connections are airtight. (Taping connections helps maintain an airtight seal.)	Prevents air from entering the system and clients intrapleural space. Thus, maintains negative pressure in the system.
c. Three-bottle system:	
■ Obtain drainage collection, water-seal, and suction-control bottles.	Suction increases the negative pressure gradient between the intrapleural space and the drainage system by evacuating air from the bottles, thus maintaining a constant, higher level of negative pressure.
■ Connect drainage and water-seal bottles as stated in the Two-bottle system, Step d.	Maintains integrity of the water-seal by collecting drainage in the first bottle.
■ Pour sterile water or saline into water-seal bottle so the straw tip is submerged 2 cm (1 in).	Maintains water-seal, preventing air from reentering the intrapleural space.

Steps	Rationale
■ Pour sterile water or saline into the suction control bottle. Physician is responsible for determining fluid level in the suction control bottle. It is usually set at 20 cm (7.9 in).	Fluid level in this bottle dictates the highest amount of negative pressure that can be present within the system, i.e., 20 cm of water is approximately −20 cm of water pressure. Any additional negative pressure applied to the system will be vented into the atmosphere through the suction-control rod. This safety device prevents damage to pleural tissues from an unexpected surge of negative pressure from the suction source.
■ Connect suction tubing from the suction-control bottle to the suction source.	While fluid level controls the maximum amount of negative pressure, the suction source establishes the minimum amount of effective negative pressure in the system. A constant, gentle bubbling in the suction-control bottle indicates that adequate negative pressure is being maintained (Erickson, 1981a).
■ Tape all connections in the system.	Maintains an airtight seal within the system.
■ Check system for patency by: Clamping the drainage tubing that will connect the client to the system. Connecting tubing from the suction-control bottle to the suction source. Turning on the suction source to the prescribed level.	Provides a chance to ensure an airtight system before connecting it to the client. Allows correction or replacement of system if it is defective before connecting it to the client. *Note:* Bubbling will be seen from the water-seal at first because there is air in the tubing and system initially. This should stop after a few min unless there are other sources of air entering the system. If bubbling continues, check connections and locate source of the air leak as described in Table 5.

Table 5 Problem solving with chest tubes

Problem	Solution
Air leak:	Locate leak:
Continuous bubbling in the water-seal bottle/chamber, indicating leak is between client and the water-seal.	Tighten loose connections between client and water-seal. Loose connections cause air to enter the system. Leaks are corrected when constant bubbling stops.
Bubbling continues, indicating the air leak has not been corrected.	Cross-clamp chest tube close to client's chest. If bubbling stops, the air leak is inside the client's thorax (client-centered) or at the chest tube insertion site (Palau and Jones, 1986). *Unclamp tube and notify physician immediately.* Reinforce chest dressing. Leaving chest tube clamped with a client-centered leak can cause collapse of the lung, mediastinal shift, and eventual collapse of the other lung from the buildup of air pressure within the pleural cavity.
Bubbling continues, indicating leak is not client-centered.	Gradually move clamps down the drainage tubing away from the client and toward the suction-control chamber, moving one clamp at a time. When bubbling stops, leak is in the section of tubing or connection that is in between the two clamps. Replace tubing or secure connection and release clamps (Erickson, 1981b).

Bubbling continues, indicating leak is not in the tubing.

Leak is in the drainage system. Change drainage system (Erickson, 1981b; Palau and Jones, 1986).

Determine that chest tubes *are not clamped, kinked, or occluded.* Obstructed chest tubes trap air in the intrapleural space when there is a client-centered air leak.

Notify physician immediately.

Tension pneumothorax:
Severe respiratory distress.
Chest pain.
Absence of breath sounds on affected side.
Hyperresonance on affected side.
Mediastinal shift to unaffected side.
Tracheal shift to unaffected side.
Hypotension.
Tachycardia.

Prepare immediately for another chest tube insertion; obtain a flutter (Heimlich) valve or large-gauge needle for short-term emergency release of air in the intrapleural space; have emergency equipment, e.g., oxygen and code cart, near the client.

Dependent loops of drainage tubing have trapped fluid.

Drain tubing contents into drainage bottle. Coil excess tubing on mattress and secure in place.

Water-seal is disconnected.
Water-seal bottle is broken.

Connect water-seal and tape connection.

Insert distal end of water-seal straw into sterile solution so that the tip is 2 cm below surface level (Carroll, 1986) and set up a new water-seal bottle. If no sterile solution is available, double clamp the chest tube while preparing a new bottle.

Water-seal straw is no longer submerged in sterile fluid.

Add sterile solution to the water-seal bottle until the distal tip is 2 cm under surface level (Erickson, 1981b); *or* set the water-seal bottle upright so that the tip is submerged.

Steps	Rationale
■ Turn off suction source and unclamp drainage tubing before connecting client to to the system.	Having the system connected to suction when it is initiated could cause damage to pleural tissues from sudden increase in negative pressure. The suction source is turned on again after the client is connected to the three-bottle system.
d. Disposable Commercial Drainage System: ■ Remove sterile wrapping.	Maintains sterility of the system. The system is packaged in this manner so it can be used under sterile operating room conditions (Carroll, 1986).
■ While maintaining sterility of the drainage tubing, stand the system upright and add sterile water or saline to the appropriate chambers: 1. For a two-bottle system (without suction), add sterile solution to the water-seal chamber, (second chamber) bringing fluid to the required level as indicated. 2. For a three-bottle system (with suction), add sterile solution to the water-seal chamber (second chamber) as described above and an amount of sterile solution (prescribed by	The same system can be used as either a two- or three-bottle system depending upon the chambers used. Maintains water-seal, preventing air from reentering the intrapleural space. Fluid drains from the chest into the first chamber. Maintains water-seal and establishes maximum amount of negative pressure that can be exerted in the system. Turning up the suction source causes more vigorous bubbling in the suction-control chamber, but does not increase the amount of negative pressure exerted on the pleura (Carroll, 1986). Fluid drains from the chest into the first chamber.

Steps	Rationale
physician) to the suction-control chamber, usually 20 cm (7.9 in).	
■ If ordered, connect suction tubing to the suction source.	Maintains minimum amount of effective negative pressure in the system. This is indicated by a constant gentle bubbling in the suction control chamber (Erickson, 1981a).
■ Check system for patency (see Three-bottle system)	Provides a chance to ensure an airtight system before connecting it to the client.
■ Tape all connections in the system.	Provides an airtight seal within the system.
6. Position the client:	Permits optimal drainage or fluid and/or air.
a. Semi-Fowler's to high Fowler's position to evacuate air (pneumothorax).	Air rises to the highest point in the chest. Pneumothorax tubes are usually placed on the anterior aspect at the midclavicular line, second or third intercostal space (Carroll, 1986).
b. High Fowler's position to drain fluid (hemothorax).	Permits optimal drainage of fluid. Posterior tubes are placed on the midaxillary line, eighth or ninth intercostal space.
7. Wash hands.	Reduces transmission of microorganisms.
8. Administer parenteral premedications, such as sedatives, analgesics as ordered.	Reduces client anxiety and pain during procedure.
9. Assist physician in providing psychological support to the client. a. Reinforce preprocedure explanation. b. Instruct client throughout procedure.	Reduces client anxiety and assists in efficient completion of procedure.

Steps	Rationale
10. Show anesthetic to physician.	Allows physician to read label of drug before administering it to client.
11. Hold anesthetic solution bottle upside down with label facing physician.	Allows physician to withdraw solution properly while maintaining surgical asepsis.
12. Assist physician to attach drainage tube to chest tube.	Connects drainage system and suction (if ordered) to the chest tube.
13. Tape the tube connection between the chest and drainage tubes.	Secures chest tube to drainage system and reduces risk of air leaks causing breaks in the airtight system.
14. Check patency of air vents in system:	
a. Water-seal vent must be without occlusion.	Permits the displaced air to pass into the atmosphere.
b. Suction-control chamber vent must be without occlusion, when using suction.	Provides safety factor of releasing excess negative pressure into the atmosphere.
15. Coil excess tubing on mattress next to the client. Secure with a rubber band and safety pin or the system's clamp.	Prevents excess tubing from hanging over the edge of the mattress in a dependent loop. Drainage could collect in the loop and occlude the drainage system.
16. Adjust tubing to hand in a straight line from top of the mattress to the drainage chamber.	Promotes drainage.
17. If the chest tube is draining fluid, indicate the time (e.g., 0900) that drainage was begun on the drainage bottle's adhesive tape of a bottle setup, or on the write-on surface of a disposable commercial system.	Provides a baseline for continuous assessment of the type and quantity of drainage.

Steps	Rationale
18. Strip or milk chest tube only if indicated: a. Postoperative mediastinal chest tubes are manipulated if nursing assessment indicates an obstruction of drainage secondary to clots or debris in the tubing. b. Postoperative assessment is done every 15 minutes for the first 2 hours. This assessment interval then changes *based on client's status.*	Stripping is controversial and should be performed only if hospital policy permits and there is a physician's order (Krauss, 1985; Johanson, 1988). Stripping creates a high degree of negative pressure and has potential of pulling lung tissue into drainage holes of the chest tube (Duncan and Erickson, 1982; Duncan, Erickson, and Weigel, 1987).
19. Provide 2 shodded hemostats for each chest tube. Shodded hemostats are usually attached to the top of the client's bed with adhesive tape or clamped to client's clothing during ambulation.	Chest tubes are only clamped under specific circumstances: a. To assess for an air leak (see Table 5). b. To empty or change the collection bottle or chamber (Farley, 1988). This procedure is performed only by physician or nurse who has received training in the procedure. c. To change disposable systems (Erickson, 1981b). Have new system ready to be connected before clamping the tube, so that transfer can be rapid and the drainage system reestablished. d. To change a broken water-seal bottle in the event that there is no sterile solution container available.

Steps	Rationale
	e. To assess if client is ready to have chest tube removed. This is done by physician's order (Farley, 1988). In this situation, nurse must monitor client for the recreation of a pneumothorax (see Table 5).
20. Assist client to a comfortable position.	Reduces client anxiety and promotes cooperation.
21. Dispose of used, soiled equipment.	Prevents accidents involving contaminated equipment.
22. Wash hands.	Reduces spread of microorganisms.
23. Record procedure and client's cardiopulmonary assessment.	Documents procedure and client response.

Nurse Alert

Client with a hemothorax, who is also on anticoagulants, may need to have anticoagulant therapy reduced or discontinued until the hemothorax is resolved or controlled.

Teaching Considerations

Teach clients and families to:
- Inform the nurse of increased chest pain or difficult breathing.
- Never lift drainage system higher than the chest tube insertion site.
- Notify nurse immediately if a bottle breaks.
- Keep system upright at all times.
- Prevent pulling on the chest tube.
- Notify nurse immediately if there are changes in the way the system is functioning.

Applying a Nasal Cannula

A nasal cannula is a simple device that can be inserted into the nares for delivery of oxygen and that allows the client to breathe through his mouth or nose. It is available for all age groups and is adequate for both short- and long-term use in the hospital or at home.

Potential Nursing Diagnoses

Impaired gas exchange related to decreased lung expansion
Impaired gas exchange related to inadequate oxygen intake
Impaired gas exchange related to airway secretions

Equipment

Nasal cannula
Oxygen tubing
Humidifier
Oxygen source with flowmeter
"No smoking" signs

Steps	Rationale
1. Wash hands	Reduces transmission of micro-organisms.
2. Attach cannula to oxygen tubing.	Establishes connection with oxygen source. Oxygen tubing has extension length so client has some mobility.

Steps	Rationale
3. Adjust oxygen flow to prescribed rate, usually between 1 and 6 L/min. Observe that water in humidifier is bubbling.	Administers oxygen at prescribed rate. Oxygen flow rates greater than 6 L/min do not increase oxygen concentration but do irritate nasal mucosa, causing swallowing of gas and abdominal distention.
4. Place prongs of cannula in client's nose and adjust band to client's comfort. (Fig. 172)	Reduces chance that client will remove cannula because of discomfort.

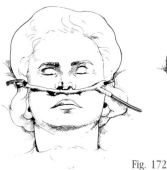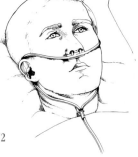

Fig. 172

5. Check cannula every 8 hours.	Patency of cannula and oxygen flow are ensured.
6. Keep humidification jar filled at all times.	Inhalation of dehumidified oxygen is prevented.
7. Assess client's nares, external nose, and ears for mucosal and/or skin breakdown every 6-8 hours.	Prolonged use of nasal oxygen can increase risk of mucosal breakdown in nares. Tape can irritate bridge of nose. Elastic band can excoriate ears.
8. Check oxygen flow rate and physician's orders every 8 hours.	Delivery of prescribed oxygen flow rate is ensured.
9. Record in client's record time that therapy was initiated, oxygen flow rate, route of administration, and client's response.	Documents that procedure was performed.

Nurse Alert

In clients with underlying obstructive lung disease the flow rate of oxygen should not exceed 2 L/min. Higher rates can depress the stimulus to breathe.

Client Teaching

Clients may be placed on home oxygen via nasal cannula. They and their families must then be taught the hazards of oxygen therapy, the rationale for it, the correct flow rate, and the proper use and cleaning of oxygen equipment.

Pediatric Considerations

In general, oxygen is delivered via an oxygen tent to a child.

Geriatric Considerations

Frail elderly clients are at increased risk of skin breakdown resulting from the placement of an oxygen cannula. The sites for skin breakdown include the nares and ears. Skin breakdown can be minimized by frequent assessment of and care to these areas.

Cardiopulmonary Resuscitation (Two Nurses)

The purpose of cardiopulmonary resuscitation (CPR) is to restore an airway, breathing, and circulation to a client who has sustained catastrophic disruption of these functions.

Cardiopulmonary arrest is characterized by an absence of pulse and respirations and by dilated pupils. CPR is a basic emergency procedure for life support, consisting of artificial respiration and manual external cardiac massage.

Potential Nursing Diagnoses

Decreased cardiac output related to absence or irregularity of heartbeat

Impaired gas exchange related to inadequate respirations

Impaired tissue perfusion related to absence or irregularity of heartbeat

Equipment

Oral airway if immediately available

Automatic manual breathing unit (AMBU) bag if immediately available

Steps	Rationale
1. Determine if person is unconscious by shaking him or shouting at him: "Are you OK?"	Confirms that person is unconscious as opposed to intoxicated, sleeping, or hearing impaired.
2. Determine presence of carotid pulse and respirations.	Presence of pulse *and* respiration contraindicates initiation of CPR.

Steps	Rationale
3. Call for assistance, seek help from passerby, call for additional nurses. Goals of care: restore airway, breathing, circulation.	One person cannot maintain CPR indefinitely. Without relief, rescuer fatigues, chest compressions are ineffective, and volume of air ventilated into victim's lungs decreases.
4. Place victim on hard surface such as floor, ground, or backboard.	External compression of heart is facilitated. Heart is compressed between sternum and hard surface.
5. Place yourself in correct position, which is also somewhat comfortable:	You may be administering CPR for extended period, particularly in community setting. Correct comfortable position decreases skeletal muscle fatigue.
a. *Two-person rescue:* One person faces victim, kneeling parallel to victim's head. Second person moves to opposite side and faces victim, kneels parallel to victim's sternum.	Allows one rescuer to maintain breathing while other maintains circulation, without getting in each other's way.
6. Restore open airway: a. *Head tilt-chin lift* (Fig. 173): Elevate chin with one hand and apply downward pressure on forehead until teeth are almost together but mouth is still open.	Airway obstruction from tongue is relieved. If necessary, remove foreign body.

Fig. 173

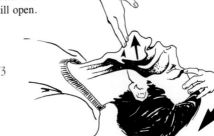

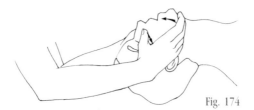

Fig. 174

Steps	Rationale
b. *Jaw thrust maneuver* (Fig. 174) can be used by health professionals but is not taught to general public. Grasp angles of victim's lower jaw and lift with both hands, displacing the mandible forward while tilting the head backward.	Jaw thrust maneuver should be used whenever cervical neck injury is suspected. This permits opening of airway without manipulating spinal column.
7. If readily available, insert oral airway.	Maintains tongue on anterior floor of mouth and prevents obstruction of posterior airway by tongue.
8. Administer artificial respiration:	
a. Mouth-to-mouth:	
■ *Adult:* Pinch victim's nose and occlude mouth with yours. Blow 2 full breaths into victim's mouth (each breath should take 1-1.5 seconds); allow victim to exhale between breaths.	Airtight seal is formed and air is prevented from escaping from nose. Hyperventilation is promoted and assists in maintaining adequate blood oxygen levels. In most adults this volume is 800 ml and is sufficient to make the chest rise. An excess of air volume and fast inspiratory flow rates are likely to cause pharyngeal pressures that exceed esophageal opening pressures, allowing air to enter the stom-

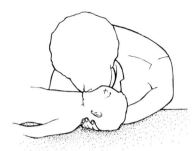

Fig. 175

Steps	Rationale
	ach and result in gastric distention, thereby increasing the risk of vomiting.
■ *Child:* Place your mouth over child's nose and mouth (Fig. 175) For mouth-to-mouth resuscitation of child, administer two slow breaths lasting 1 to 1 ½ seconds with a pause in between.	Airtight seal is formed and air is prevented from escaping from nose. Because an infant's air passages are smaller with resistance to flow quite high, it is difficult to make recommendations about the force or volume of the rescue breaths. However, three factors should be remembered: (1) rescue breaths are the single most important maneuver in assisting a nonbreathing child, (2) an appropriate volume is one that makes the chest rise and fall, and (3) slow breaths provide an adequate volume at the lowest possible pressure, thereby reducing the risk of gastric distention.
b. AMBU:	
■ *Adult and child:* For AMBU bag resuscitation use proper size face mask and apply it under chin, up and over victim's mouth and nose (Fig. 176).	Airtight seal is formed as bag is compressed and oxygen enters client.

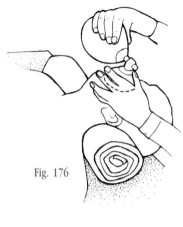

Fig. 176

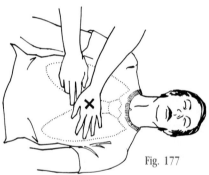

Fig. 177

Steps	Rationale
9. Observe for rise and fall of chest wall with each respiration. If lungs do not inflate, reposition head and neck and check for visible airway obstruction, such as vomitus.	Ensures that artificial respirations are entering lungs.
10. Suction secretions if necessary or turn victim's head to one side.	Suctioning prevents airway obstruction. Turning client's head to one side allows gravity to drain secretions.

Steps	Rationale
11. Assess for presence of carotid pulse (adults) or brachial pulse (infants).	Carotid artery pulse will persist when the more peripheral pulses are no longer palpable. Performing external cardiac compressions on a victim who has a pulse may result in serious medical complications.
12. If pulse is absent, initiate chest compressions: a. Assume correct hand position: ■ *Adult:* Place hands 1-2 cm above xiphoid process on sternum. Keep hands parallel to chest and fingers above chest. Interlocking fingers is helpful. Extend arms and lock elbows. Maintain arms straight and shoulders directly over victim's sternum. (Fig. 177)	Places hands and fingers over heart in proper position. Prevents xiphoid process and rib fracture, which can further compromise cardiopulmonary status. (Fig. 178)

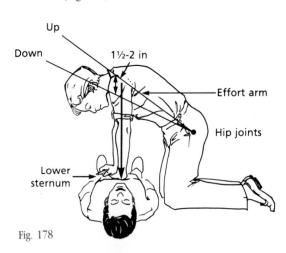

Fig. 178

Steps   Rationale

- *Child:* Place finger
  tips of index and mid-
  dle fingers of 1 hand
  1-2 cm above xiphoid
  process. Fingers
  should be on the ster-
  num at the level of
  the nipples.
- *Infant:* Place thumbs
  together on sternum
  with fingers extending
  around ribs. (Fig. 179)

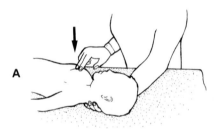

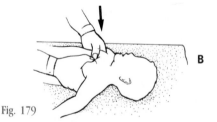

Fig. 179

b. Compress sternum to   Compression occurs only on
   proper depth from   sternum. Pressure necessary for
   shoulders. Do not rock.   external compression is created
   - Adult and adolescent: by nurse's upper arm muscle
     4-5 cm (1.5-2 in)   strength.

Steps	Rationale
■ Older child: 3-4 cm (1-1.5 in).	
■ Toddler and preschooler: 2-4 cm (0.75-1.5 in).	
■ Infant: 1-2 cm (0.5-1 in).	
NOTE: Ratio of compressions to breaths for two rescuers is 5 to 1. One rescuer is 15 to 2.	
c. Maintain proper rate of compression:	Proper number of compressions/min should be delivered to ensure adequate cardiac output.
■ Adult and adolescent: 80/min (count one 1000; two 1000).	
■ Older child, 80-100/min.	
■ Toddler and infant: 100-200/min.	
d. Continue mouth-to-mouth or AMBU ventilations.	Adequate ventilations promoted.
■ Adult and adolescent: every 5 seconds (12/min).	
■ Older child: every 4 seconds (15/min).	
■ Infant and toddler: every 3 seconds (20/min).	
13. Palpate for carotid pulse with each external chest compression for first full minute. If carotid pulse is not palpable, compressions are not strong enough.	Assessment of pulse validates that adequate stroke volume is achieved with each compression.
14. Continue CPR until relieved or until victim regains spontaneous pulse and respirations.	Artificial cardiopulmonary function is maintained.

Nurse Alert

If CPR must be interrupted, the interruption should not last longer than 5 to 30 seconds. CPR is interrupted when changing personnel, during defibrillation, or when transporting the victim. The nurse should remind rescue team members of the number of seconds elapsing.

FLUIDS

Venipuncture

Venipuncture is a technique in which a vein is punctured transcutaneously by a sharp rigid stylet (such as with a butterfly needle, an angiocatheter, a needle attached to a syringe, or a Vacutainer). The general purposes of venipuncture are to collect blood, instill a medication, start an intravenous infusion, or inject a radiopaque substance for x-ray examination of a body part or system. The present skill deals with obtaining a blood specimen. Skill 13-2 discusses venipuncture for the purpose of initiating an intravenous infusion.

Nursing Diagnoses

Potential for injury related to venipuncture
Potential alteration in skin integrity
Anxiety related to impending venipuncture
Pain related to venipuncture

Equipment

Disposable gloves
Specimen tubes
Alcohol and Betadine (povidone-iodine) cleaning swabs
Rubber tourniquet
Towel to place under client's arm
Sterile gauze pads (2 × 2)
Band-Aid or adhesive tape

Syringe method
Sterile needles (20 to 21 gauge for adult; 23 to 25 gauge for child)
Sterile syringe of appropriate size

Vacutainer method
Vacutainer tube with needle holder
Sterile double-ended needles

Steps	Rationale
1. Wash hands.	Reduces transmission of micro-organisms.
2. Apply disposable gloves.	Reduces transmission of blood-borne pathogens. Gloves should be worn when handling items soiled by body fluids (CDC, 1987).
3. Gather all equipment needed and bring to client.	Maintains organization and avoids having to leave client while you get more equipment.
4. Close bedside curtain or room door.	Provides for client's privacy.
5. Organize equipment on clutter-free surface.	Reduces risk of contamination and accidents.
6. Assist client to supine or semi-Fowler position with his arm extended straight. Place small towel under upper arm.	Stabilizes client's arm and provides easy access to venipuncture site.
7. Open sterile packages using sterile technique.	Prevents contamination of sterile objects.
8. Select distal site in vein to be used. Veins frequently used for blood sampling include those in antecubital fossa and those in lower arm.	If sclerosing or other damage occurs to vein, proximal site in same vein is still usable.
9. If possible, place client's arm in dependent position.	Permits venous dilation, thereby improving visability of vein.
10. Place tourniquet 5-15 cm (2-6 inches) above venipuncture site. Encircle client's arm and pull one end of tourniquet tightly over other, looping one end under other. Do not use a knot.	Allows vein to distend with blood, for better visibility. Permits quick release of tourniquet with one hand.
11. Palpate distal pulse below tourniquet.	Pressure from tourniquet should not impede arterial flow.

Steps	Rationale
12. Select well-dilated vein. It may help to have client make fist. Do not keep tourniquet on longer than 1-2 minutes.	Muscle contraction increases venous distention. Prolonged tourniquet time may cause venous stasis and thereby alter test results.
13. Clean venipuncture site with povidone-iodine (Betadine) solution and follow with alcohol. Move in circular motion out from site approximately 5 cm (2 inches).	Betadine is a topical anti-infective; alcohol, a topical antiseptic. Together these agents reduce skin surface bacteria.
14. Remove needle cover from syringe or Vacutainer and inform client that he is about to feel a stick.	Client has better control over his anxiety when he knows what to expect.
15. Place thumb or forefinger of your nondominant hand 2.5 cm (1 inch) below site and pull client's skin taut toward you.	Stabilizes vein and prevents rolling during needle insertion.
16. Hold syringe or Vacutainer and needle at 15- to 30-degree angle from client's arm with bevel of needle up.	Reduces chance of penetrating both sides of vein during insertion. Bevel up causes less trauma to vein.
17. Slowly insert needle into vein.	Prevents puncture of entire vein.
18. With syringe, pull back gently on plunger while securing barrel. Hold Vacutainer securely and advance specimen tube into needle of holder.	Secure hold on syringe or Vacutainer prevents needle from advancing. Pulling on syringe plunger or inserting tube creates vacuum needed to draw blood into syringe or Vacutainer.
19. Note flow of blood into syringe or tube.	If blood fails to appear, indicates that needle is not in vein or vacuum has been lost in specimen tube.

Steps	Rationale
20. Obtain desired amount of blood.	Test results are more accurate when specified amount is drawn.
21. Once specimen obtained, release tourniquet.	Reduces bleeding at site when needle is withdrawn.
22. Remove needle from vein: Place gauze 2 × 2 or alcohol pad over venipuncture site without applying pressure. Using other hand, withdraw needle by pulling straight back from venipuncture site.	Pressure over needle can cause discomfort. Straight removal of needle from vein prevents injury to vein and other surrounding tissues.
23. Apply pressure to site.	Pressure controls bleeding. If client has been anticoagulated, pressure may be necessary for 3-5 minutes to prevent hematoma formation.
24. For blood obtained by syringe, transfer specimen to tube. Insert needle through stopper of blood tube and allow vacuum to fill tube. Do not force.	Vacuum present in specimen tube causes blood to enter. Forcing blood into tube can cause hemolysis.
25. For blood tubes containing additives, gently rotate back and forth 8-10 times.	Additives mixed to prevent clotting.
26. Inspect puncture site for bleeding and apply Band-Aid.	Keeps puncture site clean and controls final oozing.
27. Attach properly completed identification label to each tube, affix requisition, and send to lab.	Tests should be performed properly. Incorrect labeling can cause diagnostic error.
28. Dispose of needles, syringes, soiled equipment and wash hands.	Reduces transmission of microorganisms.

Nurse Alert

Pressure must be applied to the venipuncture site in clients with a bleeding disorder or low platelet count or in those receiving anticoagulant therapy. It will decrease the risk of hematoma formation.

Client Teaching

If a woman has impaired lymphatic drainage (as may occur following a mastectomy), she should be instructed to tell care givers to avoid blood sampling from that arm. Impaired lymphatic drainage results in edema, and venipuncture in that extremity is difficult. Lack of lymphatic flow also predisposes the client to infection from skin puncture.

Pediatric Considerations

The nurse should not make numerous punctures in a child's arm for blood sampling. This can be extremely upsetting. A young child who requires venous sampling may need restraining by a staff member or parent. This will help immobilize the limb and prevent sudden movement that could result in serious injury to the blood vessel.

Geriatric Considerations

A frail elderly client's veins are fragile, and venipuncture becomes more difficult. The nurse should carefully assess such a client before venipuncture so he does not have to be repeatedly stuck with the needle. Because the elderly client's veins are fragile, bleeding may occur more easily in the tissues once the needle is withdrawn.

Initiating Intravenous Therapy

Venipuncture is a technique in which a vein is punctured transcutaneously by a sharp rigid stylet, such as an angiocatheter, or by a needle attached to a syringe. The major use of this technique is to initiate and maintain intravenous fluid therapy. In many settings the nurse has primary responsibility for initiating intravenous therapy with an angiocatheter.

Potential Nursing Diagnoses

Actual or potential fluid volume deficit related to prolonged vomiting, diarrhea, burns, or restricted intake
Anxiety related to impending needle stick
Pain related to needle stick

Equipment

Correct solution
Infusion set
Intravenous tubing to deliver prescribed rate
Angiocatheter
Alcohol and povidone-iodine (Betadine) cleaning swabs
Tourniquet
Disposable gloves
Arm board
2 × 2 gauze and Betadine ointment
Tape that is cut and ready to use
Towel to place under client's hand
Intravenous pole
Razor (optional)

Steps	Rationale
1. Wash hands.	Reduces transmission of micro-organisms.
2. Gather all equipment needed and bring it to bed-side.	Maintains organization and avoids having to leave client to get more equipment. More than one of each piece of equipment is recommended in case a piece of sterile equipment becomes contaminated.
3. Organize equipment on clutter-free bedside stand or over-bed table.	Reduces risk of contamination and accidents.
4. Open sterile packages using aseptic technique.	Prevents contamination of sterile objects.
5. Check IV solution, using "five rights." Make sure that any prescribed additives (e.g., potassium or vitamins) have been added.	IV solutions are medications and should be double-checked at this point to reduce error.
■ NOTE: When using bottled intravenous solution, remove metal cap and metal and rubber disks beneath cap.	Permits entry of infusion tubing into solution.
6. Have infusion set opened, maintaining sterility of both ends.	Prevents bacteria from entering infusion equipment and thus client's bloodstream.
7. Place roller clamp 2-4 cm (1-2 inches) below drip chamber.	Proximity of roller clamp to drip chamber allows more accurate regulation of flow rate.
8. Move roller clamp up to *off* position. (Fig. 180)	Prevents accidental spillage of intravenous fluid on you, client, bed, or floor.
9. Insert infusion set into fluid bag:	

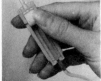

Fig. 180

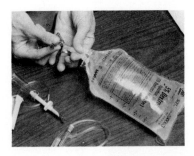

Fig. 181

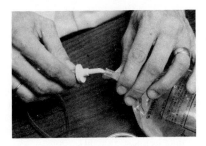

Fig. 182

Steps	Rationale
■ Remove protective cover from intravenous bag without touching opening. (Fig. 181)	Maintains sterility of solution.
■ Remove protector cap from insertion spike, not touching spike, and insert spike into opening of intravenous bag. (Fig. 182))	Prevents contamination of solution from contaminated insertion spike.
■ Be sure that insertion spike is completely inserted into opening of intravenous bag. (Fig.183)	Permits spike to puncture membrane at end of intravenous bag opening, thereby allowing fluid to flow from bag into tubing.

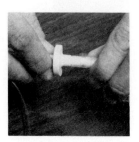

Fig. 183

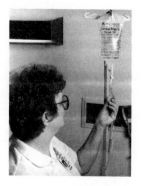

Fig. 184

Steps	Rationale
10. Fill infusion tubing:	
■ Compress drip chamber and release.	Creates suction effect, and fluid enters drip chamber.
■ Remove needle protector and release roller clamp to allow fluid to travel from drip chamber through needle adapter. Return roller clamp to *off* position. (Fig. 184)	Removes air from tubing and permits it to fill with solution.
■ Check tubing for air bubbles. If present, remove them by allowing more fluid to flow through tubing. Collect excess solution in basin and discard.	Large air bubbles can act as emboli.
■ Replace needle protector.	Maintains sterility of system.
11. Apply disposable gloves.	Reduces transmission of blood-borne pathogens. Gloves should be worn when handling items soiled by body fluids (CDC, 1987).
12. Select appropriate angiocatheter for venipuncture.	Size and type of needle depend on type of fluid to be infused and expected duration of therapy.

Steps	Rationale
13. Select distal site in vein to be used.	If sclerosing or other damage to vein occurs, proximal site in same vein is still usable.
14. If large amount of body hair is present at insertion site, shave it off.	Reduces risk of contamination from bacteria that may be present on hair. Also makes removal of adhesive tape less painful.
15. If possible, place extremity in dependent position.	Permits dilation and visability of vein.
16. Place tourniquet 10-12 cm (5-6 inches) above insertion site. Tourniquet should obstruct venous, not arterial flow. (Fig. 185)	Diminished arterial flow prevents venous filling. Check for pressure of the distal pulse.
■ NOTE: Do not tie tourniquet in a knot; use a loop tie.	Permits quick release of the tourniquet with one hand.

Fig. 185

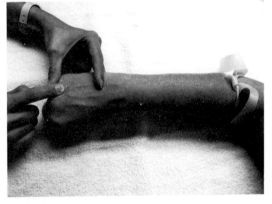

Steps	Rationale
17. Select well-dilated vein. May help to have client make fist.	Muscle contraction increases venous distention.
■ NOTE: Be sure that needle adapter end of infusion set is nearby and on sterile gauze or towel.	Permits smooth quick connection of infusion tubing to the intravenous needle.

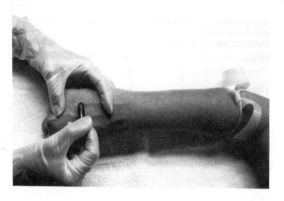

Fig. 186

Steps	Rationale
18. Clean insertion site with providone-iodine (Betadine) solution, followed by alcohol. Move in circular motion out from site 5 cm (2 inches). (Fig. 186)	Betadine is topical anti-infective; alcohol is topical antiseptic. Together these agents reduce skin surface bacteria.
19. Puncture vein using needle. Place needle at 30-degree angle with bevel up about 1 cm (½ inch) distal to actual site of venipuncture. Insert angiocatheter bevel-side up at 30-degree angle distal to actual site of venipuncture. (Figs. 187-188)	Allows you to place needle parallel with vein. Thus, when vein is punctured, risk of complete penetration is reduced.
20. Look for blood return through angiocatheter, indicating that needle has entered vein. Remove needle from angiocatheter, leaving catheter in place. (Fig. 189)	Increased venous pressure from tourniquet increases backflow of blood into catheter or tubing. Small flexible catheter remains to permit entry of intravenous fluids.

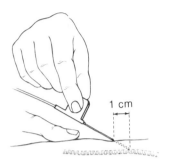

Fig. 187

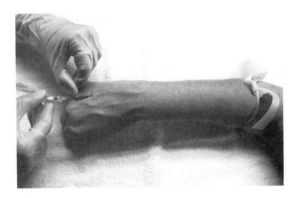

Fig. 188

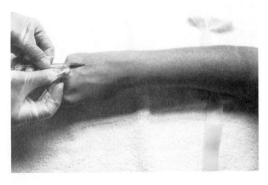

Fig. 189

Steps	Rationale
21. Connect needle adapter of infusion set to hub of an-giocatheter. To maintain sterility, do not touch entry point of needle adapter or hub of angiocatheter.	Prompt connection of infusion set maintains patency of vein.
22. Stabilizing catheter with one hand, release tourni-quet with other. Begin IV at ordered rate.	Permits venous flow. This pre-vents clotting in vein and ob-struction of flow of solution.
23. Secure IV catheter or nee-dle.	
a. Place narrow piece (½ in) of tape under cathe-ter, and cross tape over catheter.	
b. Place povidone-iodine solution at venipuncture site. (Fig. 190)	Solution ointment is topical an-tiseptic germicide that reduces bacteria on skin and decreases risk of local or systemic infec-tion. When transparent dressing is used, povidone-iodine solu-tion is recommended; ointment interferes with adherence of dressing to skin.

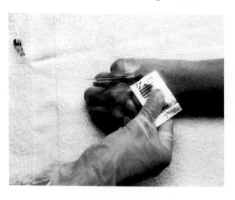

Fig. 190

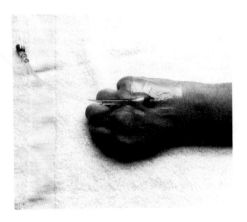

Fig. 191

Steps	Rationale
c. Place second piece of narrow tape directly across catheter.	
d. Place transparent dressing over venipuncture site, following manufacturer's directions. (Fig. 191)	
e. Secure infusion tubing to catheter with piece of 1-inch tape.	Further stabilizes connection of infusion to catheter.
24. Begin infusion.	Maintains patency of IV line.
25. Note date and time of placement of intravenous line. Dressing should be changed according to manufacturer's directions.	Reduces bacteria in infusion tubing and on client's skin.
26. Record in nurse's notes type of fluid, insertion site, and type of catheter or needle used at time infusion began.	Documents that procedure was performed.

Nurse Alert

Venipuncture is contraindicated in a site that shows signs of infection, infiltration, or thrombosis. Infection is indicated by redness, tenderness, swelling, and warmth. Infiltration is identified by localized edema, blanching, and coolness of the surrounding tissues. Thrombosis is indicated by pain, swelling, and inflammation along the vein. To avoid displacement of the angiocatheter, an arm board is used.

Client Teaching

Clients and their families should be instructed not to move the extremity with the angiocatheter in place. Excessive motion can cause the angiocatheter to become displaced, resulting in an infiltration.

Pediatric Considerations

The nurse should not make numerous punctures in a child's arm for blood sampling. This can be extremely upsetting. A young child may need to be restrained to prevent infiltration and disruption of the intravenous flow rate.

Geriatric Considerations

The veins of elderly persons may be fragile, and consequently venipuncture is more difficult. In addition, frail elderly clients are at risk of infiltration and thrombosis due to irritation of the walls of the vein.

Regulating Intravenous Flow Rates

Once an intravenous infusion is in place and secured, the nurse has the responsibility of regulating its rate according to physician's orders. An infusion rate that is too slow can lead to further cardiovascular and circulatory collapse in a client who is dehydrated, in shock, or critically ill. A too rapid infusion rate can result in fluid overload. The nurse calculates the infusion rate to prevent incorrect fluid administration.

Potential Nursing Diagnoses

Potential fluid volume deficit related to inaccurate IV flow rate
Potential fluid volume excess related to inaccurate IV flow rate

Equipment

Paper and pencil
Watch with second hand

Steps	Rationale
1. Read physician's orders and follow "five rights" to be sure that you have correct solution and proper additives.	IV fluids are medications; following the "five rights" decreases chance of medication error.
2. Intravenous fluids are usually ordered for 24-hour period, indicating how long each liter of fluid should run. For example: Bottle 1—1000 ml D5W c̄ 20 mEq KCl 8 AM-4 PM	Determines volume of fluid that should infuse hourly.

Steps	Rationale

Bottle 2—1000 ml D5W c̄
20 mEq KCl
4 PM-12 MN
Bottle 3—1000 ml D5W c̄
20 mEq KCl
12 MN-8 AM
Total 24-hour IV intake:
3000 ml

3. To determine hourly rate, divide volume by hours:

$$\frac{3000 \text{ ml}}{24} = 125 \text{ ml/hr}$$

Provides even infusion over 24 hours.

4. Intravenous fluid orders for 24-hour period may also be written as:
   Bottle 1—1000 ml D5W c̄
   20 mEq KCl 8
   AM-4 PM
   Bottle 2—1000 D5W c̄ 20
   mEq KCl
   4 PM-12 MN
   Bottle 3—500 D5W
   12 MN-8 AM
   Hourly rate would be:

Fluid needs vary. Rate must be as ordered.

$$\frac{2000}{16} = 125 \text{ ml}$$ (8 AM-12 MN)

$$\frac{500}{8} = 63 \text{ ml}$$ (12 MN-8 AM)

5. Once hourly rate has been determined, minute rate is calculated based on drop factor of infusion set. Minidrip or microdrip infusion set has drop factor of 60 drops (gtt) per milliliter. Regular drip or macrodrip infusion set has drop factor of 15 gtt/ml

Allows you to calculate hourly flow rate based on this formula:

$$\frac{\text{Total volume} \times \text{Drop factor}}{\text{Infusion time in minutes}}$$

Steps	Rationale
6. Using formula, calculate minute flow rates: Bottle 1 (1000 ml c̄ 20 mEq KCl) *Microdrip* $$\frac{125 \text{ ml} \times 60 \text{ gtt/ml}}{60 \text{ minutes}}$$ $$= \frac{7500 \text{ gtt}}{60 \text{ min}}$$ $= 125$ gtt/min *Macrodrip* $$\frac{125 \text{ ml} \times 15 \text{ gtt/ml}}{60 \text{ minutes}}$$ $= 31\text{-}32$ gtt/min	Volume is divided by time.
7. Time the flow rate by counting drops in drip chamber for 1 minute by watch, then adjust roller clamp to increase or decrease speed of infusion. Check this rate hourly. (Figs. 192, 193)	Determines if fluids are being administered too slowly or too fast.

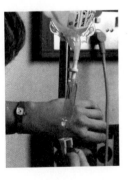

Fig. 192

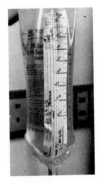

Fig. 193

Steps	Rationale
8. Place adhesive tape on intravenous bag next to volume markings. This figure is based on 125 ml in 8-hour period.	Time taping of intravenous bag gives you visual cue as to whether fluids are being administered at proper rate.

Steps	Rationale
9. Record in nurse's notes if IV is patent and infusing on time.	Documents IV status and client's response.

Nurse Alert

An IV that fails to infuse on time may be an early sign of infiltration. If an infusion pump is used, the nurse should still monitor the rate of flow of the intravenous solution at least hourly. If intravenous fluids are excessively slow or fast, the physician should be contacted for revision of the intravenous flow rate before the flow is increased or decreased.

Client Teaching

The client should be instructed to report any tenderness or swelling at the venipuncture site.

Pediatric Considerations

Intravenous flows in children should always be maintained at the prescribed rate because fluid imbalances can occur rapidly. Pediatric settings usually require that infusion pumps or volume control devices be used with intravenous therapy.

Changing Intravenous
Infusion Dressing

The nurse changes intravenous solutions using sterile technique to discontinue a specific solution or to remove an empty solution container and reconnect the tubing to a new container.

Potential Nursing Diagnoses

Potential for infection related to contaminated dressing

Equipment

Correct intravenous solution (or D5W to maintain patency of IV line)
Roller clamps
IV pole and bag

Steps	Rationale
1. Wash hands.	Reduces transmission of micro-organisms.
2. Have next intravenous solution prepared at least 1 hour before it is needed. If solution is prepared in pharmacy, be sure that it has been delivered to floor. Check that it is correct and properly labeled.	Prevents finding empty intravenous bag without having replacement bag. Also prevents medication error.
3. Prepare to change solution when it remains in neck of bag or bottle.	Prevents air from entering intravenous tubing and vein from clotting due to lack of intravenous flow.
4. Be sure that drip chamber is half full.	Provides intravenous fluid while bag is being changed.

Steps	Rationale
5. Prepare new solution for hanging: ■ Plastic bag—Remove protective cover from entry site. ■ Glass bottle—Remove metal cap, metal disk, and rubber disk.	Permits quick, smooth, and organized change from old solution to new.
6. Move roller clamp to reduce flow rate.	Prevents solution remaining in drip chamber from emptying.
7. Remove old solution bag or bottle from intravenous pole.	Brings work to eye level.
8. Quickly remove spike from old container and, without touching tip, insert it in new container.	Reduces risk that solution in drip chamber (Step 3) will run dry. Also maintains sterility.
9. Hang new bag.	Allows gravity to assist with delivery of fluid.
10. Check for air in tubing.	Reduces risk of embolus.
11. Make sure that drip chamber contains solution.	Reduces risk that air will enter tubing.
12. Regulate flow rate as prescribed.	Maintains measures to restore fluid balance.
13. Record in nurse's notes amount and type of fluid infused and amount and type of new fluid.	Documents that solution has infused and new infusion has been started.
14. Stabilize hub of intravenous catheter or needle. Gently pull out old tubing. Maintaining stability of hub, insert needle adapter of new tubing into hub.	Prevents accidental displacement of catheter or needle.
15. Open roller clamp.	Permits new intravenous solution to enter catheter or needle.
16. Apply new dressing.	Reduces risk of bacterial infection from skin.

Steps	Rationale
17. Regulate intravenous drip according to physician's orders.	Maintains fluid and electrolyte balance.
18. Record in nurse's notes changing of tubing and solution.	Documents that measures to maintain sterility were carried out.
19. Wash your hands.	Reduces transmission of microorganisms.

Nurse Alert

An intravenous tubing change is easier if the nurse organizes it to occur when a new solution bag is being hung. There are times, however, when it is not possible to have the two procedures occur simultaneously, as when tubing is accidentally punctured with a needle.

Irrigating a Heparin Lock

A heparin lock is an IV needle with a small "well" covered by a rubber diaphragm (Fig. 194). This device decreases costs by reducing the need for continuous IV therapy with client's who require only IV medications and not fluids. In addition, a heparin lock increases the client's mobility, safety, and comfort.

When clients have heparin locks, the lock must be flushed on a routine basis and after IV medications. Flushing of the heparin maintains patency of the cannulated vein. (Policies may differ from agency to agency as to the frequency of irrigation and the irrigant used.) This skill focuses on the irrigation of the heparin lock.

Potential Nursing Diagnoses

Pain related to venipuncture
Potential for infection related to irrigation procedure

Equipment

Heparin flush solution: 1 ml/100 units or 1 ml/10 units*
Sterile normal saline vial*
Medication ticket, card, or form
Prepared medication
2 3-ml syringes used for heparin or saline flush
25-gauge needles to attach to syringes to irrigate heparin lock
Antiseptic swab
Watch with second hand—used for timing of IV bolus or IV piggyback medication

*Irrigation solution varies from agency to agency.

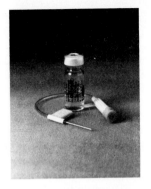

Fig. 194

Steps	Rationale
1. Wash hands.	Reduces transmission of micro-organisms.
2. Verify physician's order and prepare medication.	Ensures that proper medication is given to the right client.
3. After preparing medication, apply small-gauge needle to syringe.	Used to insert through IV line or heparin lock.
4. Check client's identification by looking at armband and asking full name. Compare with medication ticket.	Ensures drug is administered to correct client.
5. Flush heparin lock a. Heparin only ■ Prepare a syringe with 1 ml of heparin flush solution. ■ Prepare a syringe with 1 ml of normal saline. Attach 25-gauge needle to syringe.	Flush solution keeps heparin lock patent after drug is administered. Used to assess for blood return in heparin lock.
b. Saline only: ■ Prepare 2 syringes with 2 ml of normal saline each. Attach 25-gauge needle to each syringe.	Normal saline has been found to be effective in keeping intravenous locks patent.

Steps	Rationale

c. Heparin and saline:

- Clean the lock's rubber diaphragm with the antiseptic swab.

  Cleaning prevents introduction of microorganisms during needle insertion.

- Insert needle of syringe containing normal saline through center of diaphragm. Pull back gently on syringe plunger and look for blood return.

  Determines if IV needle or catheter is positioned in vein. (At times a heparin lock will not yield a blood return even though lock is patent.)

- Flush reservoir with 1 cc saline by pushing slowly on the plunger.

  Cleans needle and reservoir of blood.

- Remove needle and saline-filled syringe.

- Clean the lock's diaphragm with the antiseptic swab.

  Prevents transmission of infection.

- Insert the needle of syringe containing prepared medication through center of diaphragm.

  Using center of diaphragm prevents leakage.

- Inject medication bolus slowly over several min. (Each medication has a recommended rate for bolus administration. Check package directions.) Use a watch to time the administration.

  Rapid injection of an intravenous drug can kill a client.

- After administering the bolus, withdraw the syringe.

- Clean the lock's diaphragm with an antiseptic swab.

  Prevents transmission of infection.

Steps	Rationale
d. Heparin flush: ■ Insert needle of syringe containing the heparin through the diaphragm. Inject 1 ml heparin slowly, then remove syringe.	Maintains patency of needle by inhibiting clot formation. Diluted heparin avoids anticoagulation.
e. Saline flush: ■ If using only saline to flush the reservoir, inject 2 cc of saline after each use of the intravenous lock.	
6. Wash hands.	Reduces transmission of microorganisms.
7. Dispose of uncapped needles and syringes in proper container	Prevents accidental needle sticks.
8. Record patency of heparin lock, drug, dosage, route, irrigation of heparin lock procedure, and assessment of venipuncture site.	Accurate documentation reduces risk of future medication errors. Provides data for ongoing assessment of heparin lock system.

Nurse Alert

Be sure to loosen tape or dressing over IV site in order to see it clearly before administering drug.

Administering a Blood Transfusion

Blood products are ordered by the physician to restore circulatory blood volume, improve hemoglobin, or correct serum protein levels. The administration of blood or blood components is a nursing procedure.

Potential Nursing Diagnoses

Actual or potential fluid volume deficit related to loss of blood volume

Equipment

In addition to that used to initiate an IV infusion
Normal saline IV solution, 0.9%
Infusion set with inline filter
Large catheter (18 or 19 gauge)
Correct blood product
Another nurse to double-check correct blood product with correct client
Disposable gloves

Steps	Rationale
1. Wash hands.	Reduces transmission of micro-organisms.
2. Apply disposable gloves.	Reduces transmission of blood-borne pathogens. Gloves should be worn when handling items soiled by body fluids (CDC, 1987).